DODGING
DEMENTIA

DODGING DEMENTIA

Understanding MCI and other risk factors

MARY JORDAN

WITH A CHAPTER BY DR JERRY THOMPSON

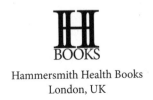

Hammersmith Health Books
London, UK

First published in 2024 by Hammersmith Health Books
– an imprint of Hammersmith Books Limited
4/4A Bloomsbury Square, London WC1A 2RP, UK
www.hammersmithbooks.co.uk

British Library Cataloguing in Publication Data: A CIP record of this book is available from the British Library.

Print ISBN 978-1-78161-242-2
Ebook ISBN 978-1-78161-243-9

Commissioning editor: Georgina Bentliff
Typeset by: Julie Bennett of Bespoke Publishing, UK
Cover design by: Madeline Meckiffe
Cover image by: © Overearth/John T Takai/Shutterstock
Index: Dr Lawrence Errington
Production: Deborah Wehner of Moatvale Press Ltd
Printed and bound by: TJ Books, Cornwall, UK

Contents

Contents

Introduction

Dementia is an umbrella term for various symptoms such as short-term memory loss, perceived personality change and impaired intellectual functions. This may include impaired judgement, difficulties with abstract thinking and loss of communication skills. This book is about avoiding dementia whatever its cause, but it principally refers to dementia caused by Alzheimer's disease, vascular changes to the brain (vascular dementia), Lewy body dementia and fronto-temporal dementia.

The terms 'dementia' and 'Alzheimer's disease' are often confused, particularly in articles written by the popular press, but it is important to remember that Alzheimer's disease is just one of the diseases that causes symptoms of dementia. Sometimes in this book the term 'Alzheimer's disease' is used when quoting from a particular piece of research because that is the term used in that research, but in general the book discusses the avoidance of dementia – that is the avoidance of the collection of symptoms mentioned above.

When I wrote the first edition of this book in 2012, the mere suggestion of 'avoiding dementia' was an almost outrageous idea. At the time no one knew what caused these symptoms and therefore it seemed that it was impossible to do anything about avoiding developing it.

We know a lot more about the condition today and we have more information about how to treat some forms – for example, there is better treatment for vascular dementia – but in truth we still do not know what causes most forms of dementia. Research now is leaning towards the suggestion that there is no one cause – rather there any many predisposing factors and that it is the accumulation of a number of life incidents, lifestyle choices and genetic factors that allow the symptoms of dementia to develop. Medical opinion is that once these symptoms manifest and the onset of brain degeneration is established (usually by the evidence of a brain scan), there is a 'cascade' effect and that dementia can only get worse. A contrary opinion is held by those who have faith in the Bredesen protocol (see Chapter 4) and its ability to turn the tide. However, this book is primarily concerned with the avoidance of dementia – that is, taking steps to reduce the risk of developing any of the symptoms in the first place.

In 2020 a special report by the renowned research journal, *The Lancet*, listed 12 factors that could be modified and that might prevent or at least delay up to 40% of dementias.[2] We will examine all these factors but, in addition, this book will discuss other risk factors for which there is no research-based specific evidence but which are strongly indicated to be relevant. At times I have drawn on my own experience gained as a result of working for 15 years with people who have dementia.

The *Lancet* report makes specific recommendations and it is wise to look at these in detail. We should always remember, though, that current medical knowledge is just that – current knowledge – and that medical discoveries can change treatments overnight. As an example, we can take Semmelweis's findings that gastric ulcers resulted from a bacterial (Helicobacter) infection. Previously it was thought that stress or certain foods were the cause. Current recommendations are also subject to popular thinking and to pressure exerted by professional bodies. Consider how smoking advice has changed.

Mild cognitive impairment (MCI)

Since at present we do not have a definitive causal factor for dementia, then it is worth examining various opinions and discussing their relevance. Of particular relevance is the increasing tendency for people who are worried about cognitive symptoms (such as memory loss, difficulty in forward planning and organisation, and problems with communication) to be 'diagnosed' with 'mild cognitive impairment' (MCI). MCI is not an actual illness and therefore I use the term 'diagnosed' with caution and only here because of the number of people who have told me that, after consulting their doctor, mild cognitive impairment has been given as a diagnosis.

MCI is considered to be simply a descriptive term for slight impairments in brain function (such as memory, planning, and attention span) which do not actually prevent the person carrying out the functions of everyday living. People who have MCI *are* able to carry out those functions and to live independently and manage ordinary everyday activities. They may find it harder to do these things and they may take longer to plan an event or come to a decision, but they are not unable to carry out everyday functions.

In this book we examine the increased risk of developing dementia if we have MCI, but it needs to be remembered that not everyone with MCI goes on to develop dementia. With awareness of the general and personal risk factors described in this book, you can lower the risks and improve your chances of 'dodging dementia' whatever your starting point.

How to use this book

There are three Parts to this book.

In Part I we look at some of the many possible causes of dementia, including examining various research papers which highlight these possible causes. I have also highlighted some of my own experience of working with people with MCI and dementia; this experience is not necessarily backed up by research but I think it may be of interest to readers and it is based on observation of many diagnosed cases and discussion with colleagues over a number of years. Observations based on my experience rather than research are clearly identified.

In Part II, the emphasis is on assessment of individual risk. Although some readers will be health professionals, I have assumed that there will also be many who are reading this book because they are concerned about the possibility of themselves developing dementia (and even a health professional might fall into this category). I have also tried to show ways that you can do a personal assessment of your own risk of developing dementia. There is no 'tick list' as such because – despite what the popular press often suggest – there is no easy way to define your overall risk. Rather, Part II allows you to look at your own personal situation and identify where you might need to make lifestyle changes.

In Part III, I examine these lifestyle changes in more detail. Many of them are very easy to make. Others may be tough, especially where addictions are involved. It comes down to personal choice and the importance to you personally of lowering your risk.

Living with uncertainty

The most important thing for me to emphasise is that we still do not know the actual 'cause' of dementia. We know a lot more than when I wrote the first edition, and fresh research is showing us new evidence almost daily as well as new areas of interest. But reading this book can only take you so far. You may choose not to make any changes to your lifestyle, or to the medication you take, and to 'leave things to chance'. You may consider that your personal risk of developing dementia is very small. Even if you take all the steps outlined to reduce your risk, you may still find yourself in a few years' time hearing that you have the 'dreaded diagnosis'.

However, most of us do take sensible precautions against risk. We wear a helmet when cycling or riding, we fasten our seat belt when driving in the car, we wear eye protection when using DIY or gardening equipment. Taking the precautions against the known risks of dementia is not such a strange step. It is also worth noting that some of the precautions against these risks really are very easy to implement.

I look forward to the day when we can really suggest that we have found the cause (or causes) of dementia and need no longer live in fear of developing it.

PART I

What do we know?
Risk factors for dementia

Chapter 1

Age, personality and social factors

- The brain changes with age but dementia is not a natural result of ageing.
- Variety in life, in social contacts and in leisure pursuits all seem to be significant protective factors.
- Level of education seems to have some bearing on risk of developing dementia.
- Brain plasticity and cognitive reserve may also influence risk.

This chapter looks at some very basic factors that research indicates may be associated with an increased risk of dementia. The first of these is age. We hear so often that cases of dementia are increasing because we are living longer, but is this really the case?

Age and dementia

Whilst there are some quite striking examples of younger people developing dementia (particularly 'familial' dementia, which is examined on page 124), the most prominent 'risk factor' for developing the condition is indeed age. Dementia is a disease of older people. However, it is not an inevitable result of ageing. Many older people have excellent cognition, even taking into account the natural slowing down of life in general as we get older.

A person's risk of developing dementia rises from one in 14 over the age of 65, to one in six over the age of 80. That is, one in 14 people over the age of 65 have dementia.[1] Also, that five in six people over the age of 80 do not. What makes the difference between those who do have dementia symptoms and those who don't? Let's examine some of the factors that seem to play a part alongside age. Strikingly, research shows that personality and social factors are significant in this respect.

Personality, social factors and dementia

The Nun Study

David Snowdon, a US-based neurologist, has studied ageing and dementia in a population of 678 nuns. 'The Nun study', as it is known, is a most useful source for researchers because it is a longitudinal study (that's a study that follows a group over a long period of time) of ageing and Alzheimer's disease, which began in 1986 as a pilot study on ageing and disability. It started out using data collected from the older School Sisters of Notre Dame living in Mankato, Minnesota, but later expanded to include older Notre Dame Sisters living in the midwestern, eastern and southern regions of the United States. Participants in the Nun Study include women representing a wide range of functioning and health. Some Sisters are in their 90s; others may be in their 70s. Some are highly functional, with full-time jobs; others are severely disabled, unable to communicate, possibly even bed-bound.

Each of the 678 participants in the Nun Study agreed to participate in annual assessments of their cognitive and physical function. The assessments have included medical examinations and giving blood samples, and many of the nuns agreed to donate their brains after death for research. This means that the Nun Study represents the largest brain-donor population in the world. In addition, the Sisters have given investigators full access to their convent and medical records.

The study has found that traits in early, mid and late life have strong relationships with the risk of Alzheimer's disease, as well as the mental and cognitive disabilities of old age. For example, among the documents reviewed as a part of the study were autobiographical essays that had been written by the nuns upon joining the Sisterhood. It was found that an essay's lack of complexity, vivacity and fluency was a significant predictor of its author's increased risk for developing Alzheimer's disease in old age. Roughly 80% of nuns whose writing was measured as lacking in 'linguistic density' went on to develop Alzheimer's disease in old age; meanwhile, of those whose writing was *not* lacking, only 10% later developed the disease.[2]

Social engagement

From personal experience of supporting clients with dementia, I have frequently noted the number who have told me, 'I am not particularly sociable'. Another factor of note is the number of people who develop dementia shortly after retiring from full-time employment. It seems that in many cases the work in which they were involved was a significant factor in giving meaning to their life and it may have been the main social involvement that they had with others.

> **Covid-19 note:** The isolation caused by the Covid lockdowns and difficulties with social interaction have, in many cases it appears, brought incipient dementia out into the open. It is difficult to tell whether such dementia might have been delayed if the social isolation had not been enforced or whether possibly it might never have manifested itself at all.

Research findings on personality

The suggestion that certain personality 'types' might be more prone to developing dementia has been studied elsewhere. A paper by Nicholas and colleagues, published in 2010, detailed the results of a case-control study which set out to examine whether personality traits and social networks were significant to the risk of developing Alzheimer's disease (AD) specifically.[3] This study examined 217 individuals diagnosed with probable late-onset AD (160 women and 57 men). For the purposes of this study, 'informants' who had lived with or were in regular contact with the people studied (the 'subjects') were asked to provide retrospective information about the personality of subjects and controls. The controls were recruited from the same population area and were mostly unaffected siblings of the subjects. The informants were asked to remember the subject they knew as she/he had been in their 40s. The subjects were, at the time of the research, aged between 61 and 98 years. Additional assessments were made about social activity when subjects had been in their 40s, and also the level of physical and mental challenge they would have experienced at that time. Cases and controls were also assessed for major depressive episodes and/or abnormal anxiety prior to the age of 50.

The results showed that a selection of abnormal personality traits was over-represented in those diagnosed with AD. The AD group had a significantly greater number of personality disorder traits compared with the control group. A high correlation was found particularly with what are classed as 'cluster-A personality traits' (paranoid, schizoid and schizotypal) and a lesser but significant correlation with 'dissocial', 'borderline', 'histrionic' and 'narcissistic' traits (all precise psychological terms). In some cases, the differences were particularly striking between those with AD and the controls (for example, some of those who later developed AD had few close friends, found difficulty in enjoying close friendships, bore more grudges, preferred solitary activity, had difficulty expressing feelings and were easily offended). Those people with AD also had sparser social networks than the controls.[3]

The researchers accepted that the main limitation of the study was that they employed a retrospective rating of personality and social activity so the findings may have been subject to recall bias. However, they concluded that: 'There is an association between abnormal personality traits and AD. Individuals with AD also appear to have had lower levels of social interactivity.'

Long-term v. short-term personality traits

It is sometimes difficult to distinguish whether apparent personality traits are part of a long history or whether a solitary lifestyle and unwillingness to embrace new experiences are the result of recent life events. Doctors sometimes use a system of asking those closest to the person with dementia to describe his/her personality 10 years previously in order to assess how his/her personality traits might have changed. Of course, this is a very inexact method, relying as it does on memory which may be tainted by past life events and the particular relationship of the relative with the person being assessed. For example, if the person giving the assessment is a son or daughter of the patient, then their whole concept of the parent's personality may be coloured by their experiences of that person when they were children. Conversely, if they are now in mid-life they may have only vague memories of their parent's personality 10 years previously as they might have been living apart and heavily involved with their own young family.

Several questionnaires have been developed to make this assessment, but even the health professionals using them will admit their weakness and lack of objectivity.

Covid-19 note: People who were excessively frightened by the media with reference to Covid-19 and who therefore hid themselves away and avoided contact even with close friends and family may appear to be socially isolated but this can be due to recent events rather than being a matter of normal personality.

Is personality fixed or fluid?

There is evidence that the brain is affected by the clinical beginnings of dementia up to 25 years before dementia manifests itself in an obvious way. The brain appears to have a vast 'spare' capacity and it may be that, as evidence seems to indicate, a higher neural reserve delays the onset of clinical signs. What this might mean is that the changes in attitude, activity and what we call 'personality' may begin many years before overt evidence of dementia so that we are once again brought up against the 'which came first?' question.

The study of personality has a long history. 'Personologists' make much of the innate organisation of personality and believe that behaviour is consistent over time and in different situations. Others ('situationists' or 'behaviourists') assert that the environment and situation may change how we behave. A third view is that of 'interactionists', who believe that people constantly adjust their behaviour according to situations and the society in which they find themselves.

Recently, personality psychologists have come to agree on personality traits known as the 'five factor model' consisting of five major personality factors: neuroticism, extraversion, openness, agreeableness and conscientiousness. This model is now so well accepted that any member of the general public can undertake a 'personality test' via the internet and be given scores for these five traits.

In greater detail, the five factors of personality are thought to be as follows:

Neuroticism is the tendency to experience unpleasant emotions easily, particularly emotions such as anger, anxiety, embarrassment and guilt. Neuroticism also refers to the degree of emotional stability and control of impulses.

Extraversion refers to outgoingness, sociability and the tendency to seek the company of others.

Openness refers to intellectual curiosity and willingness to seek new experiences, to appreciate art, to be open to new ideas and to enjoy variety. Sometimes this factor is called 'intellect'.

Agreeableness refers to the tendency to be cooperative, trustful and compassionate in contrast to being antagonistic and suspicious of others.

Conscientiousness refers to being orderly, dutiful and self-disciplined.

What most personality studies have demonstrated is that personality does in fact remain stable over time. Some investigations have extended into old age,[4, 5] and these studies agree with the stability of personality. Where changes tend to occur, they are in agreeableness, which increases, and in extraversion, which declines. In plain words, this might indicate that elderly people become more tolerant but less inclined to socialise.

Personality changes in dementia

Researchers Ann Kolanowski and Ann Whall looked at the notion of personality in dementia in a paper published in the *Journal of Nursing Scholarship*.[6] This paper examined personality traits in persons who had been diagnosed with dementia. As the authors showed, research seems to indicate that certain patterns of aberrant behaviour in people with dementia are common according to what has happened to them in the past. This paper also suggested that the personalities of people with dementia 'reflect adaptive patterns that have served them in the past'.

Generally it seems that when someone has dementia, their base-line personal traits do not change; their personality reflects the pattern of their past personality as regards the five factors. So someone who was introverted and suspicious of others before they developed dementia is not likely to suddenly become outgoing and friendly as a result of their dementia. They are more likely to become more introverted and more suspicious of others. Someone who was generally friendly and trusting will probably remain friendly and trusting.

What often happens, and what carers and relatives often cite as the first signs of a 'change in personality', is that someone who had a previously absorbing hobby stops taking part in or attending to this hobby. In a similar vein, someone who frequently attended social events and took a full part in them begins to shun going out or, whilst continuing to attend events, takes a less and less active part. Whilst this may seem to be a change in personality trait it is actually the result of the deterioration in the brain.

The frontal lobe of the brain contains several parts, which all act together to form the 'executive' or 'management' centre. The executive centre is responsible for planning actions and learning new tasks and for motivation and impetus. When this part of the brain is affected, people can lose their 'get up and go', becoming lethargic and unable to perform even regular activities which gave pleasure and satisfaction in the past. It may also be true that someone who is becoming aware that their memory and abilities are failing may try to avoid going into situations where they feel under stress through having to remember names and faces or taking part in conversations which they may have trouble following.

Social interaction and networking

Research cited above also took account of social activity and social networks.[3] A 1999 paper by Bassuk and colleagues published in the *Annals of Internal Medicine* examined the relationship between social disengagement and the incidence of cognitive decline in elderly people living in the community.[7] Altogether, 2812 elderly people aged over 65 were interviewed and followed up over several years. Their level of social interaction was assessed by taking account of such things as having a spouse, monthly visual contact with three or more relatives or friends, yearly non-visual contact with 10 or more relatives or friends, attendance at religious services, group membership, and regular social activities. Compared with people who had five or six social ties, those who had none were at increased risk for 'incident cognitive decline'. The researchers concluded that lack of a good social network is a risk factor for cognitive impairment among elderly people.[7] These conclusions were similar to those drawn in the study by Nicholas and colleagues.[3]

The six dimensions of wellness

Another study, published in the *Journal of Holistic Nursing* took this further and defined 'the six dimensions of wellness' which protect cognition in adults.[8] These six dimensions are defined as follows:

1. **occupational**, meaning the ability to contribute to personally meaningful work in a paid or unpaid capacity.
2. **social**, meaning the ability to form and maintain positive personal and community relationships.
3. **intellectual**, meaning commitment to lifelong learning

through continuous acquisition of skills and knowledge.

4. **physical**, meaning commitment to self-care through regular participation in physical activity, healthy eating and appropriate use of health care.

5. **emotional**, meaning the ability to acknowledge personal responsibility for life decisions and their outcomes with emotional stability and positivity.

6. **spiritual**, meaning having a purpose in life and a value system.

This research looked at such things as the complexity of midlife occupation, marriage, social networks, formal education, intellectual activities, physical activity, healthy nutrition, motivational ability, purpose in life and spirituality.

The conclusions drawn were that wellness in one or more dimensions protected cognition (ability to think and understand). Cognitive benefits increased if wellness was experienced in more than one dimension. If there was a lack in any one dimension it could be compensated for by a higher degree of wellness in another. For example, wide social networks could compensate for unhappiness in one's occupation.

This concept of different dimensions of wellness might suggest why someone with a very fulfilling occupation might find that this 'compensates' for a lack of complex social networks and activities. As mentioned earlier, sometimes family members notice dementia symptoms soon after someone has retired and this theory might suggest a reason, although it would be difficult to prove.

Intelligence and education

It might seem to make sense to assume that someone who has a higher intelligence quotient (IQ) would be less likely to develop dementia but, in actual fact, a person's raw intelligence level doesn't appear to be a significant factor in determining the chance of this. However, the level of education achieved does seem to make a difference to the level of risk, along with the variety of life experiences, the breadth of social experiences and contacts and the continued pursuit of activities which expand the mind.

The exact level of education at which there is a difference in the risk of developing dementia is not really known but evidence seems to indicate that any protective factor may be due to education creating a higher 'neural reserve' (see below), which delays the onset of clinical signs. For example, education, by developing the brain, gives the brain more capacity to use in making connections, retrieving memories and using vocabulary. This means that, even when some of the brain may be degenerating due to some form of dementia, other parts of it may be called into use to 'get around' the problem.

We know that something like this happens with stroke victims. If someone has suffered a stroke, a part of their brain effectively 'dies' and is no longer of use. However, people who have had a stroke can relearn abilities they have lost. They can recover lost functions through the effect of structural changes in the surviving nerve cells in the brain (neurones) or by learning new ways to solve old problems. Put simply, people recover lost functions by 'educating' a different part of the brain to form new connections and neural pathways. (This is known as 'brain plasticity' or 'neuroplasticity'.)

It may be that if, in early dementia, a part of the brain fails to function, then a similar process takes place. It seems that someone who has benefited from more than basic education can have so developed their brain that it is able to 'get around' the problems of lost connections by changing its pathways, in the same way a motorist might use a diversion to avoid a road closure.

The conclusions of research into this are not always clear. Research results appear to show differences depending upon the type of measure of cognitive ability which was used. Where researchers used the Mini Mental Status Examination (MMSE), a commonly used test in determining the progress of dementia (see page 211), then a higher level of education appeared to show a protective effect. For example, in one research project in the USA, Constantine Lyketsos and colleagues tested a group of 1488 people on three occasions over a period of 11.5 years. They observed that more education was associated with less cognitive decline. Having at least eight years' education was associated with the maintenance of cognitive function during ageing. However, beyond nine years' education was not associated with a further reduction in cognitive decline.[9]

However, where researchers were testing individual elements of cognition, results were not always so clear cut. For example, Christensen and colleagues reported that, whilst education affected general mental status and verbal abilities (such as extent of vocabulary and similarities), it did not seem to affect speed of processing in a group of older people tested over a 3.6 year period.[10] They suggested that education had a 'compensatory' rather than a protective effect. This might tie in with the theories of brain plasticity and cognitive reserve which we will examine later in this book (see page 153).

An interesting study which mainly involved observing the effect of education in early-onset Alzheimer's disease and fronto-temporal dementia, looked at 44 people with dementia prior to age 65 years and used the number of years of formal education as a marker for cognitive reserve (see below). The findings of this study suggested that education played a role in upholding 'attentional' capacity. In other words, formal education helped those with dementia to better retain the ability to pay attention. Given that a short attention span is a major problem in early-stage dementia, this research is significant.[11]

The brain's ability to adapt

As we have seen, scientists and researchers talk about 'cognitive reserve' and 'brain plasticity'. In order to follow how this might affect the risk of dementia we need to understand these terms.

Brain plasticity

We know quite a lot about the development of the brain in infancy. In the early years, the brain develops its 'links'. A newborn's brain is only about one-quarter the size of an adult's. It grows to about 80% of adult size by 3 years of age and 90% by age 5. This growth is largely due to changes in individual neurones, which are structured much like trees. Each nerve cell begins as a tiny 'sapling' and gradually sprouts hundreds of long branches called dendrites. Brain growth is largely due to the growth of these dendrites, which serve as the receiving point for input from other neurones. Synapses are the connecting points between the axon (long tail) of one neurone and the dendrite of another. While information travels down the length of a single neurone as an electrical signal, it is transmitted across the synapse through the release of tiny packets of chemicals, or 'neurotransmitters'. On the receiving side, special receptors for neurotransmitters change the chemical signal back into an electrical signal, repeating the process in this next neurone in the chain.

The number of synapses in the cerebral cortex peaks within the first few years of life, but then declines by about one third between early childhood and adolescence.

The initial perception of an experience is generated by a subset of neurones firing together. Because they have fired together once, the neurones involved are more inclined to fire together in the future. This is known as 'potentiation' – recreating the original experience. If the same neurones fire together often, they eventually become permanently sensitised to each other so that if one fires the others do as well.

Thought processes are complex. We may describe an action in a 'straight line' fashion, but in fact each thought process involves many neurones and many synaptic connections. If one connection fails, several others may still function. Take the example of identifying a particular leaf. It grows on a tree, it is green, it rustles in the wind, it may have a name which reminds us of something else (Ivy and Holly are common girls' names and we also connect them with Christmas), it evokes a Season of the year (spring, summer, autumn or winter), it may have a scent and so on. Let us suppose that we pick up a leaf and for the moment we cannot recall what kind of a tree it comes from. It is prickly and reminds us of Christmas and the face of our little niece comes to mind. Of course – it is a holly leaf. The direct 'connection' from seeing the leaf to remembering its name momentarily failed, but by using other connections the brain has led us to the name of the leaf. Thought processes are like that.

It is believed that education enables the brain to develop its ability to make these various 'connections'. Take the simple example of the leaf again. If we lived in an oak wood and never left it, if the only trees we ever saw were oak trees and we were brought up in an environment where the only leaves we saw were oak leaves, then the first time we saw a holly leaf we might not recognise it as a leaf. Formal educational experience, and exposure to a variety of other experiences, hobbies, activities and events, together develop our ability to extend our brain connections.

Brain reserve

The idea of a 'reserve' in the brain comes from the observation scientists have made from post-mortem examinations that some people whose brains had extensive Alzheimer's disease pathology (amyloid plaques and neurofibrillary tangles), clinically had no, or very little, manifestation of the disease. Reserve is perceived as having both passive and active components. Passive components are structural features involving the anatomy of the brain. Active reserve is taken to mean the efficiency of the neural networks and the brain's ability to compensate or use alternative networks after an injury such as, for example, a stroke. Doctor Yaakov Stern in a paper entitled 'Cognitive reserve and Alzheimer's disease' suggested similarly that the concept of cognitive reserve might take two forms. In 'neural reserve' the existing brain networks are more efficient or have a greater capacity to resist damage. In 'neural compensation', other brain networks may compensate for the networks that are damaged.[12]

The scientific world is still not certain whether cognitive reserve actually prevents dementia or whether the ability to 'redirect' our brain connections just prevents the manifestation of dementia symptoms. Either way, it does not matter to the average person who is trying to dodge dementia. Since we are normally unaware of attempts by our brain to make use of 'redirections' in neural pathways, the non-appearance of signs of dementia is good enough. **As far as your neighbour is concerned, if you don't show signs of dementia you don't have dementia.**

Chapter 2

Trauma and physical and mental illness

- Illnesses and traumatic events may pre-dispose people to dementia.
- Some rare diseases may lead to dementia in their later stages.
- Type 2 diabetes is a major risk factor for cognitive dysfunction and dementia.
- Cardiac and vascular disease are important factors in vascular dementia.
- Some other diseases increase the chances of a later diagnosis of dementia.
- Some research has shown a possible infectious cause for Alzheimer's disease.
- People with dementia should be protected as far as possible from infections.

This chapter looks at possible connections between dementia and earlier adverse events – trauma (physical and/or psychological), physical illness and mental illness – and the effects these may have on the mind and body.

Trauma

Trauma can be physical, due to a blow to the head or damage to the body from, for example, a traffic accident or even a surgical procedure, or psychological, caused by repeated distress in the past, the one-off stress and horror of being involved in something like a bomb incident, or what used to be known as 'battle fatigue' and is now frequently classed as post-traumatic stress.

Few of us escape physical injury of some kind in our lives, and although not all of us have to manage severe mental health issues, we all have to deal with emotional upset, distressing happenings and the death of someone close to us – perhaps a parent, friend or sibling. Many of us also have to cope with physical or mental trauma. It may seem that, because almost no one escapes being touched by illness or trauma, this cannot be a significant factor when we are considering the cause or causes of dementia. After all, there are still many people who have suffered during their lives in many ways and yet do not exhibit the symptoms of dementia before their life's end. However, research and experience are beginning to suggest that it is not the actual experience of illness or trauma that triggers dementia but the way in which each one of us manages to deal with the experience and outcomes of these events.

Head injury

We know that trauma to the head can result in dementia either immediately or many years after the original event. In particular, we know that repeated trauma to the head, as is experienced, for example, by boxers, can result in dementia in later life. Dementia pugilistica (DP) is the neurodegenerative disease that may affect amateur or professional boxers and also athletes in other sports who suffer concussions or near concussions. The symptoms and signs of DP develop progressively over a long (apparently latent) period of, sometimes, several decades. In people with this condition, the brain changes (neurofibrillary tangles: NFTs – see page 212) associated with Alzheimer's disease are observed in very high densities in the brain. However, in Alzheimer's disease, these NFTs display different distribution patterns from those in DP. In DP a paper published in 1992 reported, NFTs were concentrated in the superficial layers of the brain's neocortex (outermost layer), whereas in Alzheimer's disease they predominated in the deep layers.[1]

DP is thought to affect around 15-20% of professional boxers. It is caused by repeated concussive blows and blows that are below the threshold of force necessary to cause concussion, or a mixture of the two. Soccer players have also been shown to be prone to develop a similar condition due to the constant 'heading' of heavy leather footballs. The replacement of leather balls with lighter synthetic materials has now made such a possibility less likely, although not impossible.

Trauma to the head resulting from injury in an accident can also result in dementia. Sometimes this occurs immediately following the accident, in which case it is clear that the trauma was responsible for the dementia. However, sometimes there appears to be a complete recovery from the head trauma but dementia develops a long time later – perhaps many years later. In this case it is not always so clear that the head injury was the cause.

There is a body of research examining a link between head injury and dementia. As an example, Plassman and colleagues published a paper investigating head injury in early adulthood and the later risk of dementia.[2] The results showed that moderate and severe head injury were linked to the development of Alzheimer's disease and dementia in general, although there was little evidence to show that minor head injury had any effect on a later risk of dementia. Since this research was based on historical records, the authors pointed out that they could not exclude the possibility that other factors were involved in the later development of dementia.

A number of studies have indicated the importance of the connection between severe head injury and the possibility of accelerated neuro-degenerative processes affecting the beta-amyloid plaques which are believed to be the root cause of dementia of the Alzheimer's type.[3, 4, 5] This body of research indicates that the head injury itself does not cause dementia at the time but that the injury seems to precipitate a degenerative process which can result in dementia at a later date. This might tic in with the current thinking that a neurological 'event' is required to trigger dementia even in the presence of the plaques and tangles generally associated with Alzheimer's disease.

A piece of research by Richard Mayeux and colleagues examined the connections between traumatic head injury and a specific gene – apolipoprotein-epsilon 4 (ApoE4). Persons who had a history of traumatic head injury and carried the ApoE4 gene had a tenfold increased risk of developing Alzheimer's disease. In this study, no increased risk of dementia was found due to head injury in those who did not carry ApoE4. This suggests that head injury might increase the risk of AD, but only through a synergistic relationship with ApoE4.[6]

These findings might help explain why not everyone who receives a moderate to severe head injury goes on to develop dementia. Most researchers are careful to point out that there are a number of indications for further research. If, for example, it could be proved that a traumatic brain injury accelerated the neurodegenerative processes underlying Alzheimer's disease, then interventions designed to block or reverse these processes could potentially be given to anyone with a head injury.

A very recent study published online, called the Protect TBI (Traumatic Brain Injury) Cohort study, suggested that three or more incidents of head injury in a lifetime are associated with significant long-term cognitive problems. This study concluded that individuals concerned should be counselled about continuing high-risk activities. The study also pointed out that concussions and severe blows to the head should be taken seriously because there might be consequences in later life.[7]

What might seem obvious is that precautions to protect oneself from head injury are extremely important. The cyclist's or climber's helmet is not just to prevent immediate death or injury but may have greater long-term benefits than at first imagined.

Hypertrophic olivary degeneration (HOD)

Hypertrophic olivary degeneration (HOD) is a rare neurological condition caused by degeneration in the brain stem, the structure that connects the brain to the spinal cord. The exact cause of this condition, which can manifest with dementia-like symptoms, is currently unknown but it is thought that trauma to the head may be a possible cause.[8]

Other forms of physical trauma

Damage to blood vessels in the brain, also known as cerebro-vascular damage, is a common biological cause of dementia. This includes strokes and/or narrowing of the blood vessels supplying the brain. Localised areas of the brain are destroyed (commonly called 'infarcts') as a result of not getting enough blood supply. Many of the same factors that cause heart disease also cause cerebrovascular disease. The type of dementia that results from cerebrovascular disease is known as vascular dementia.

It is true that in people diagnosed with vascular dementia the symptoms manifest in a different way from those diagnosed with Alzheimer's disease. In order to make a specific diagnosis, a clinician would need the results of a brain scan and a medical history (probably revealing cardiac problems or a history of stroke). However, most health professionals who are familiar with dementia would probably say that they could conclude after a meeting with someone who had dementia whether this was a vascular presentation. Vascular patients tend to react more slowly, to appear to think more slowly and to have a clear 'vascular apathy' - a slowness which can appear like a form of laziness or a reluctance to initiate action. However, they are likely to be less confused than Alzheimer's patients and, given enough time and encouragement, may be able to carry out everyday tasks adequately. Their memory may be impaired but they are more likely to be able to recall things if given clues and not stressed or hurried.

More and more doctors are coming to believe that the dividing line between Alzheimer's disease and vascular dementia is less clear cut than was formerly thought to be the case. There is a growing belief that a vascular event is required to happen in order to cause dementia even if the plaques and tangles that indicate Alzheimer's disease are present.

Mental/emotional trauma

Mental trauma has been less well researched, perhaps because it is more difficult to define. A certain amount of research has been done on the connections between post-traumatic stress disorder and dementia and mental illness in earlier life and later life dementia.

In my experience

It is rare that I meet a new dementia client who does not have a history of trauma either physical or mental. Many of my clients have had major surgery, such as open-heart procedures, hip or knee replacements and many have had multiple procedures; most would say that they have made a good recovery from the surgery. Enquiry, however, nearly always results in a mention of ongoing side effects, of further surgery necessitated by the first procedure, or of a long-term drug prescription due to the surgical operation. People seldom connect this physical trauma to the body with the onset of dementia, perhaps because dementia usually appears some years later. Researchers now know that dementia is developing years before any symptoms manifest so it seems strange that doctors themselves seldom suggest that past surgical procedures may have 'triggered' the cascade of cell death which results in the condition.

Many others amongst my clients have experienced extremely stressful or traumatic events in their lives. Of course, most people with dementia are aged over 70 years and few of us reach that age without experiencing an upsetting event, a death of a close relative or an accident of some kind. But what stands out to me is the number of clients who have gone through a very serious trauma: watching a loved one die unexpectedly, experiencing the death of a child, losing life savings in a financial 'crash', being involved in a serious motor or sports accident, going through a particularly acrimonious divorce, becoming estranged from parents or children – or multiple examples of these traumas. Events like these put a serious strain on the balance of the mind and yet no one seems to equate these traumas with a later dementia. While such adverse events may not be preventable, recognition of this vulnerability might help improve prevention.

Physical disease and dementia

It is sometimes difficult for people to understand that dementia is not a mental disease as such. Perhaps this is particularly confusing because the diagnosis of dementia is most often (though not always) made by a psychiatrist. Research also shows that, some forms of mental illness are risk factors for dementia (see below).

Alzheimer's disease, the single biggest cause of dementia, is a physical disease which affects the brain. Actual physical changes take place in the tissues of the brain which affect the way that the brain works. In the advanced stages of Alzheimer's disease the atrophy of the brain can be measured. As far as is known, it is not the result of any other disease.

Vascular dementia, currently considered to be the second most common cause of dementia, is caused by changes in the circulatory system which result in a lack of adequate blood flow to the brain. Some doctors think that a vascular 'event' such as a stroke may trigger Alzheimer's disease (see above) and that the two forms of dementia are more closely connected than was previously thought to be the case.

Though these two diseases are the most common causes of dementia symptoms, there are many other more rarely seen types which appear to develop as primary diseases.

It is also known that there are many rare physical diseases that may lead to dementia, including progressive HIV/AIDS, Creutzfeldt–Jakob disease (CJD), supranuclear palsy, Korsakoff's syndrome and Binswanger's disease. Some people with multiple sclerosis, motor neurone disease, Parkinson's disease and Huntington's disease may develop dementia as a result of the progression of their condition.

Because we are used to modern medicine being able to treat many conditions, and even to cure some of them, and because in the developed world we no longer fear the scourges of the past such as contagious diseases and disease caused by poor sanitation, there is a tendency to see illness as something which has only a short-term effect and which, after a cure has been affected, will not leave any residual problem in the human body. People have tended to become quite blasé about even very serious illness, such as pneumonia. The need to convalesce is no longer considered necessary and even taking extra rest after an illness is slightly frowned upon as 'malingering' or making a fuss.

In fact, all illness leaves its mark upon the body. People live longer now and medical practitioners are beginning to see the residual effects of illness manifesting itself in later life. For example, we now know that there is a connection between polio and symptoms of lassitude, weakness and muscle fatigue in later life, known as 'post-polio syndrome'. The viral illness chickenpox which many people contract as children, can resurface in later life as shingles, an extremely painful condition.

What we have learned from the Covid-19 outbreak: It was noted early on during the Covid-19 pandemic that people with pre-existing conditions were more likely to suffer badly from the secondary effects of the virus. Such knowledge is not new – influenza and other infections have always been more dangerous in those whose health is already compromised.

Public Health specialists acknowledged this fact and those known to have co-morbidities were contacted and asked to 'shield' during the pandemic. The effect of this official and individual notification was to cause many to over-react and shut themselves off from society.

Media added to the over-reaction by highlighting that the elderly (meaning anyone aged over 70 years) were more vulnerable, with the result that many older people also shunned normal mixing with others, even refusing to see grandchildren for family visits. In fact, those aged over 70 years in normal health are possibly less likely to catch an infectious disease since they have some immunity built up over the years (although it is still true that older people may suffer more from secondary effects of infection).

An analysis reported in the *Journal of Social Science and Medicine* examined whether childhood illness had a long-term effect on the appearance of chronic disease in later life.[9] The authors reported that poor childhood health increased morbidity (ill health) in later life. An association with poor health in childhood was found for cancer, lung disease, cardiovascular conditions and arthritis/rheumatism. Non-infectious diseases were associated with higher rates of cancer and arthritis or rheumatism in later life, while infectious diseases were strongly associated with lung conditions such as emphysema and bronchitis. The authors stated that, 'Our results point to the importance of an integrated health care policy based on the premise of maximizing health over the entire life cycle'. Such findings do not mean that we should be anxious about trivial illness or worry about past medical history. There is, however, ample evidence for making sure that we give the body time to recover after illness and that we make every effort not to allow neglect of our health to cause problems in later life.

Dementia and chronic physical disease

We know that some illnesses, both physical and mental, and some traumatic events predispose people towards dementia in later life. Some serious diseases have already been referred to earlier in this chapter. However, there are other chronic diseases and disorders which are known to have a 'connection' with dementia. The most well documented of these are cardiac and vascular disease (including stroke) and diabetes.

Cardiovascular disease and stroke

Many people who suffer a stroke which causes temporary cognitive as well as neurological problems make a considerable if not a full recovery. They do not develop dementia and may go on to live a comfortable and active life. However, the fact is that suffering a stroke does increase your chances of developing dementia. Atrial fibrillation (a form of heart arrhythmia) in someone who has suffered an ischaemic stroke (that is a stroke due to a blocked blood vessel rather than a bleed) seems to be associated with an increased risk of developing dementia.[10]

If you have a stroke and are discovered to suffer from atrial fibrillation you will be offered medical treatment to reduce the chances of a further stroke.

Someone who has suffered a stroke will normally be subject to a number of tests and investigations to discover the ostensible cause. Health issues such as high blood pressure or cardiac disease will hopefully be addressed by the attending medical team. If you have had a stroke you can help yourself by making full use of all the physical therapy offered to you and by adopting a positive 'can do' attitude. Cognitive and physical recovery can happen over a number of months or years. The part of the brain which has effectively 'died' following the loss of blood supply will not recover (it is known as an infarct), but other parts of the brain may and frequently do take over the functions of the dead cells and remarkable recovery can be made.

There are two main types of vascular dementia known to be related to stroke:

1. **Multi-infarct dementia (MID):** Multiple, small strokes are a common cause of dementia and this is known as MID; MID occurs when blockages in the blood supply to the brain occur frequently over a period of time in the smaller blood vessels, giving rise to many tiny and widespread areas of damage. These small strokes are commonly known as transient ischaemic attacks (TIA). Often someone can suffer a TIA without any major symptoms and they may even be unaware that it has happened. Sometimes the only symptoms are fleeting, such as a few moments of dizziness or a slurring of speech which rights itself in moments or a weakness and numbness in a limb which passes off and may be put down to cramp or to sitting too long in one position. These continuing small strokes can go on for years, causing gradual loss of function and leading to confusion and intellectual deterioration. A feature of this type of vascular dementia

is that some people experience periods of relative stability before another TIA causes further significant and abrupt worsening of the symptoms.

2. **Single infarct dementia:** Sometimes a single stroke that is extremely severe or affects a particular area of the brain can cause dementia. This is called single-infarct dementia but in this case the area of damage to the brain is limited.

There is a further form of vascular dementia called sub-cortical vascular dementia (this is also known as 'small vessel disease-related dementia'). This is not caused by stroke but may be experienced by somebody who has also had a stroke. It is caused by injury to small blood vessels that are deep within the brain. The onset of this type of dementia is more gradual than stroke-related dementia, and so it appears more like the onset of Alzheimer's disease rather than the 'stepped' deterioration common to multi-infarct vascular dementia.

If you have suffered a stroke, you can make every effort to recover your physical abilities, and making adjustments to your lifestyle and co-operating with medical teams will help to prevent further strokes. This will help to preserve your cognitive abilities.

If you have been diagnosed with vascular dementia (as a result of several minor strokes/TIAs, for example) you may be given medication aimed at preventing further strokes. Treatment of vascular dementia is aimed at preventing more damage and capitalising on the cognitive abilities which are retained. Therefore the suggestions in the chapters on exercise, social and cognitive stimulation and nutrition are all relevant.

You can reduce your risk of suffering a stroke by taking regular exercise, refraining from smoking and controlling your blood pressure. You cannot usually anticipate a stroke, although there is evidence that a TIA is a serious warning sign of stroke and should not be ignored. Up to 40% of all people who have experienced a TIA will go on to have an actual stroke. Most studies show that nearly half of all strokes occur within the first two days after a TIA. Within two days after a TIA, 5% of people will have a stroke. Within three months after a TIA, 10 to 15% will have a stroke. If you believe that you have suffered a TIA you should see your doctor without delay.

Type 2 diabetes

Diabetes is a common health condition. There are 3.8 million people diagnosed with type 2 diabetes in the UK and an estimated 1 million people who have the condition but do not know it.[11]

Diabetes is the term used for a condition where the amount of glucose in the blood is too high because the body cannot metabolise it properly

There are two main types of diabetes, type 1 (often called 'juvenile onset' because it usually develops in childhood) and type 2 which is sometimes called 'maturity onset' diabetes. Type 1 diabetes develops when the insulin-producing cells in the body have been destroyed and the body is unable to produce any insulin. Type 2 diabetes develops when the body can still make some insulin, but not enough, or when the insulin that is produced does not work properly (known as insulin resistance). The following discussion is mainly concerned with type 2 diabetes.

Diabetes is a serious condition and should not be treated lightly. Uncontrolled diabetes can lead to problems with circulation which can affect the eyes, heart and peripheral parts (hands and feet).

A growing body of research links diabetes with both Alzheimer's disease and vascular dementia. There is even a school of thought which suggests that Alzheimer's disease is actually a third type of diabetes.[12] Type 2 diabetes has specifically been identified as a significant risk factor for age-related cognitive impairment, cognitive decline and dementia.[13] It has been demonstrated that people with mild cognitive impairment (MCI) who also have diabetes are three times more likely to develop dementia than those who have MCI alone.[14]

If you refer to Chapter 5 on nutritional factors and dementia, it becomes clear that the problem lies in the metabolism of glucose and the effect this has on the brain. The brain runs on glucose (although it cannot store glucose), making use of almost a quarter of the glucose and oxygen which the body takes in. Because the brain uses glucose as its main source of energy it might be thought that a high level of glucose in the blood would be good for the brain, making it work better. In actual fact, fluctuations in blood glucose level such as are caused by a diet high in carbohydrate and sugar are detrimental. The brain needs a sustained and balanced supply of glucose and this is best obtained from eating foods which cause blood glucose levels to rise more slowly and to be sustained for longer. Uncontrolled diabetes can lead to excessive high and low levels of glucose.

What does this mean in terms of dodging dementia? Firstly, the risk factors for type 2 diabetes are well known. Do not assume that because many people are developing the condition it is not serious. You should take strenuous steps to avoid becoming diabetic. Whilst some of the risk factors may not be under your control, others, like weight gain, lack of exercise and high blood pressure are likely to be within your control. Further information about risk factors is readily available on the Diabetes UK website and in their literature. Remember that, aside from the risk of dementia, type 2 diabetes increases the risk of experiencing many other health problems.

If you have been diagnosed with type 2 diabetes, you may be able to reverse the process by losing weight and addressing other health issues.[15] If this is not possible, take the condition seriously. Adjust your diet, attend for medical screening and take your doctor/diabetic nurse's advice.

Diabetics who have been diagnosed with early stage dementia need special attention from their carer to watch blood glucose levels and take medication in a timely manner.

Other physical conditions and dementia

A number of other physical conditions have been linked with dementia, especially in people known to carry the ApoE4 gene discussed earlier in this chapter in relation to head injury, but research into these is still ongoing. Information about some of these conditions and the current state of research is included here for those who are interested. It is important to remember that because we do not know the actual cause(s) of dementia some of these lines of research may later turn out not to be relevant.

Herpes simplex

At the time of writing the first edition of this book there was much publicity about a link thought to be found between Herpes simplex (the virus that causes common cold sores) and dementia. Ruth F Itzhaki from the University of Manchester did a substantial amount of research which suggested that there was evidence for a major causative role for Herpes simplex virus type 1 (HSV1), acting in combination with the APoE4 gene. However, her research, published in the *Lancet* in 1997, cautioned that: 'the combination of HSV1 in brain and carriage of an Apo-epsilon 4 allele is a strong risk factor for AD, whereas either of these features alone does not increase the risk of AD.'[16]

Newer research bears out this conclusion. A 2021 research paper concluded by stating: 'HSV1 is associated with cognitive decline but not with incident dementia in the general population. These data suggest HSV1 to be associated only with subtle cognitive disturbances but not with greater cognitive disorders that result in dementia.'[17]

Age-related macular degeneration (AMD)

Scientists have known for some time that there is a connection between AMD and Alzheimer's disease. A paper published in the *American Journal of Epidemiology* examined the relationship between AMD and Alzheimer's disease in the Rotterdam Study. The Rotterdam Study was a population-based study in the Netherlands set up to investigate factors that determine the occurrence of cardiovascular, neurological, ophthalmological, endocrine (hormone-related) and psychiatric diseases in elderly people. One of the early signs of Alzheimer's disease is the presence of extracellular senile plaques in the brain. These plaques are akin to those seen in age-related maculopathy (degeneration in the 'macular' inside the back of the eye) and they are associated with neural malfunction and cell loss. Because of these parallels, the researchers were prompted to study the appearance of the two diseases together within the Rotterdam Study. They found that people in the study who had advanced AMD when the study began showed an increased risk of developing Alzheimer's disease. The authors' conclusion was that the neural degeneration occurring in AMD and that in AD might have a common origin ('pathogenesis').[18] However, the association was only significant for the most severe stages of AMD and the authors pointed out that the association depended also on smoking and atherosclerosis.

A more recent (2019) review of all related published research (what is known as a meta-analysis) bears out these conclusions, pointing out that people with AMD have poorer cognitive function compared with controls and concluding that there is 'a significant association between dementia/AD and AMD'.[19]

Hearing impairment

Hearing impairment may seem a strange issue to associate with dementia. However, a piece of research published in 1989 found that *untreated* hearing impairment was more prevalent in those with dementia and that the risk of dementia increased with the degree of hearing loss.[20] The researchers did point out that there was no suggestion that hearing loss was a cause of dementia; rather that it might reveal or exacerbate the symptoms. Hearing impairment can cause social isolation and can also contribute to a general loss of understanding of the environment as well as, perhaps, contributing to depression. People with dementia are often reluctant to wear hearing aids even when they have been prescribed and carers sometimes find it difficult to ensure that they are worn consistently. A person who has dementia who also has severe hearing loss will be likely to be more confused if they cannot hear what is going on around them.

There is more about hearing loss and how to cope with it in Chapter 10 (page 169).

Infection

There is emerging discussion of the possibility of some forms of dementia (as well as other chronic conditions such as heart disease) resulting from infection. *Chlamydophila pneumoniae* and several types of spirochaete (a particular class of bacteria), have been suggested as possible causes.[21] Evidence to date has been inconsistent however.

Scientists at the University of Texas Medical School in Houston did some research which involved injecting brain tissue from a confirmed Alzheimer's patient into mice and compared the results with a control group. Those mice injected with the Alzheimer's brain extracts developed plaques and other alterations to the brain typical of Alzheimer's disease.[22] This research raises the possibility that some cases of Alzheimer's disease may arise from an infectious process similar to diseases like Creutzfeldt-Jakob disease – (prion diseases).

What *is* known is that infections of any kind are likely to accelerate neurodegeneration in someone who has dementia or MCI. Urinary and chest infections, in particular, are known to exacerbate symptoms in people with dementia and there is a school of thought which believes that inflammation is the prime 'culprit' in the development of the condition, particularly inflammation caused by infections. Systemic inflammation – that is, inflammation in the whole body – is known to have direct effects on brain function. Recently a number of observational studies linked the intake of non-steroidal anti-inflammatory drugs (NSAIDs – for example, ibuprofen, paracetamol) with a lowered risk of developing Alzheimer's disease,[23] and for a while this looked like a very promising research route. Unfortunately, randomised controlled trials so far have not confirmed any beneficial effect from taking NSAIDs and have pointed out that the side effects of these drugs may make things worse.[23]

There are a number of (mostly rare) infectious and inflammatory conditions which can lead to dementia; they can be treated resulting in the improvement or stability of any dementia symptoms. These diseases include Hashimoto's encephalitis, syphilis, Lyme disease (later stages) and HIV/AIDS. Usually other (non-dementia) symptoms will be evident and lead to a correct diagnosis and treatment.

Episodes of delirium, in which elderly and demented patients become extremely disoriented and confused, are frequently caused by infections, injury or surgery in these patients (see below). Urinary tract infections, which are usually caused by bacteria, appear to be particularly common inducers of psychiatric symptoms which can sometimes mimic dementia.

Post-operative cognitive impairment

Following an operation under general anaesthetic some people develop a severe (and temporary) form of confusion often termed post-operative delirium. It is known that people who suffer post-operative delirium are more likely to suffer from dementia at a later date.[24] This has been noticed more particularly in patients undergoing coronary bypass grafting.

Physical disease and dementia: Conclusion

Clearly physical disease and the risk of dementia are not unconnected. Whilst not suggesting that you should become overly concerned about minor illness, the evidence implies that as we grow older we should take care of our physical health, be sensible about minor infections or injuries and not allow minor health problems to become major ones through self-neglect. If you have a long-standing health problem you should not become blasé about the way you manage it. Whilst the human body has huge recuperative powers, you should respect the potential for future damage and protect against this as far as possible. The family and carers of people who have been diagnosed with dementia often state that they date the appearance of symptoms from a severe illness, the beginning of a physical health problem or a stay in hospital for a surgical operation.

Some doctors tend to dismiss this anecdotal evidence, suggesting that there is no robust research which proves such incidents precipitate early symptoms of dementia. Others, including consultant psychiatrists who specialise in elderly care, are more cautious. If you notice symptoms of cognitive loss following a major physical illness or surgical intervention, do not allow yourself to be dismissed as neurotic.

It is, however, important to remember that there are some physical problems – one example is a vitamin B12 deficiency, which may be associated with pernicious anaemia – which may cause memory problems and mild confusion if not treated with vitamin B12 injections. When people present to their doctor with suspected dementia, the doctor will normally conduct tests to screen out the possibility of such a cause. If you are worried about the possibility of a vitamin deficiency you can check this with your doctor (see Chapter 4 by Jerry Thomson on medication). There are also some drugs or combinations of drugs which may cause these symptoms. Sometimes the symptoms may arise even after you have been taking the drug for some time without problems. Memory loss and confusion do not always mean dementia. If you suspect a deficiency or a drug interaction, you should mention this to your doctor or pharmacist. Pharmacists are often more knowledgeable about drug interactions than GPs.

Mental illness

There are a number of links between clinical depression during adulthood and dementia in later life but it is difficult to make positive conclusions. Robert S Wilson, PhD, of Rush University Medical Center, Chicago, and colleagues, studied 917 older Catholic nuns, priests and monks who did not have dementia, beginning in 1994. Those with more symptoms of depression at the beginning of the study were more likely to develop Alzheimer's disease. For each depressive symptom registered at the beginning of the study, the risk of developing Alzheimer's disease increased by an average of 19%, and the annual rate of cognitive decline increased by an average of 24%.[25] In this study those who developed Alzheimer's disease did not show any increase in depressive symptoms before the diagnosis was made. These researchers therefore concluded that symptoms of depression might be associated with changes in the brain that reduce its resistance to dementia.

Looking at the connection another way, research reported in the *European Journal of Epidemiology* suggests that there may be a genetic link between a susceptibility to depression and a higher than normal risk of dementia.[26] In this study of 6596 subjects, researchers looked at the association of self-reported depression which required treatment by a psychiatrist, to family history of psychiatric disease, dementia and Parkinson's disease. Not surprisingly perhaps, a family history of psychiatric disease was significantly associated with overall depression. In addition, people who had two or more first-degree relatives, such as parents, siblings or children, with dementia, had a higher risk of depression. Those with only one relative with dementia had no increased risk. The researchers suggested that their findings indicated that there might be 'shared susceptibility gene(s) underlying these diseases'. Of course it might be concluded that the stress of caring for two or more relatives with dementia could be a cause of depression.

Depression and additionally bipolar disorder are also identified with a higher than average risk of dementia in another piece of research which looked at all hospital admissions with primary affective disorder (low mood and depression) in Denmark during the period 1970–1999. A total of 18,726 patients with depressive disorder and 4248 patients with bipolar disorder were included in the study.

Risk of a later diagnosis of dementia was significantly increased according to the number of times patients had been admitted to hospital previously. It was concluded that every admission for depression increased the possibility of later dementia by 13% and every admission for bipolar disorder increased the possibility of dementia by 6%. The researchers concluded that the risk of later dementia increased with the number of episodes of hospitalisation with depression.[27] This is not an easy conclusion to interpret, however. Is one to conclude that hospital admission makes dementia more likely or that a more severe experience of bipolar (therefore involving hospital admission) is the risk factor?

Mood disorders in general may be risk factors for the development of dementia. A study involving 455 people with mood disorders including major depression and bipolar disorder compared these patients with 1003 'normal' controls and showed that cognitive decline developed faster in people with mood disorders after the age of 65 than in the control group.[28] The authors concluded that not only might depression in later life be an early manifestation of dementia but that those who develop depression or fail to recover from an earlier depression may have a higher risk of developing dementia. The researchers did, however, point out that the results could equally show that changes resulting from past disease or injury might cause both mood disorders and dementia.

This sample of the research into a possible causal effect of dementia in connection with depression indicates both the difficulties which researchers encounter and the lack of robust conclusions from research to date. The only clear conclusion appears to be that there is some connection between clinical depression and a later diagnosis of dementia. Clinicians also know that people diagnosed with dementia are often also depressed.

An important point to note is that some of the medications for severe depression and bipolar disorder may cause memory problems and mild confusion. These problems are linked to the medication and should be addressed by the doctor prescribing it. They are not, in themselves, indications of developing dementia.

Autism/Asperger syndrome

People who care for someone with dementia often report a lack of empathy as one of the first noticeable symptoms. Carers who have a relative or friend with autism or Asperger syndrome sometimes note that the lack of empathy and inability to sympathise or seem to understand the concerns of others has similarities with the behaviours of those with autism/Asperger's.

DK Sokol and colleagues in their research paper on autism, Alzheimer's disease and fragile X syndrome highlight the genes which are implicated in both autism and Alzheimer's disease.[29] Some more recent research has also highlighted several connections between these two disorders, including the possible role played by electromagnetic smog (see Chapter 10, page 168).[30]

Although some researchers are convinced of a link between

the two conditions, more research is needed, especially where adults with autism are followed up over time. It is now known, however, that autistic adults have an increased risk of dementia, and a likelihood of verbal memory difficulties and long-term (as opposed to short-term) problems with memory retrieval.[31]

Conclusion

In this chapter we have looked at trauma and various acute and chronic conditions which are believed to be risk factors for the development of dementia. In Chapter 3 we will be looking at lifestyle factors which may play a part in raising the risk of dementia. Whereas illness and trauma may be unavoidable, it is in the area of lifestyle change that we can each choose to make a difference.

Chapter 3

Lifestyle choices, miscellaneous factors and risk of dementia

- Some lifestyle choices may increase the risk of developing dementia in later life.
- Physical exercise and a full social life are considered to be key to reducing risk.
- Smoking increases the risk of many diseases.
- The evidence about alcohol intake is equivocal.
- New evidence emphasises the need for good sleep habits.

There are a number of lifestyle choices which are thought to have a bearing on the risk of developing dementia in later life. Some, such as taking exercise and enjoying a varied social life, are discussed more fully in other chapters. In this chapter we are going to consider suggestions that have been made about the connection between the risk of developing dementia and smoking, alcohol intake, body weight, exercise, social life and sleep factors.

Let's take a brief look at exercise and social life first. These factors are considered to be of major importance and that is why they have been covered more extensively in later chapters (see pages 143 and 118 respectively).

Exercise

People are always surprised when they ask me what they can do to lower their risk of dementia and I answer 'exercise'. Everyone thinks the answer is to do 'brain exercise' – puzzles, crosswords and other conundrums – which they believe 'exercises the brain'. But it is fairly conclusively agreed by experts that doing brain puzzles only makes you better at doing brain puzzles. There are specific things you can do to extend the plasticity of the brain but it is more important to undertake physical exercise. Exercise increases the oxygen levels in the brain, improves balance, benefits the cardiovascular system and improves cognition. It has also been shown that, whilst exercise of any kind can be beneficial, the number of different types of exercise makes a difference (see Chapter 9).

People who exercise are less likely to develop dementia and this seems especially to apply to women. Light exercise is better than no exercise at all. It is clear too, that it is never too late to begin exercising. Those who already have signs of dementia or who have mild cognitive impairment (MCI) can still obtain benefit from commencing an exercise programme.

Social life

Mixing with other people, enjoying conversation, taking part in social events and feeling a part of society are all important in lowering the risk of developing dementia. Many people feel that this particular lifestyle element is strictly a matter of taste. They are happy to say that they are 'not sociable people', but social integration is important. This is not to say that you have to have a huge circle of friends and become a 'party animal' in order to lower your risk of dementia. Chapter 11 goes into more detail about the benefits of good social integration and explains how even small steps to extend your social circle can be beneficial.

Smoking

Smoking has long been considered to have a detrimental effect on health and some of the research around the effect of a regular smoking habit on cancer and heart disease is now considered to be irrefutable. The evidence for an effect of smoking on the chance of developing dementia has been more debatable. Early research seemed to indicate that smoking actually had a protective effect. This caused some concern in the medical world since at the time of this early research the indications that smoking had a detrimental effect upon health were gathering momentum.

Later research, some of which is quoted below, is considered to be more rigorous and to have more validity.

In research published in the *Lancet* in 1998, A Ott and seven colleagues conducted a population-based follow-up study of elderly people who were initially free of dementia. In this investigation, 6870 people aged 55 years and older were classified as 'never smokers' (people who had never smoked), 'former smokers' and 'current smokers'. During follow-up, all cases of dementia were recorded. The study also examined modification of risk by age, sex and the apolipoprotein E (ApoE) genotype we've discussed earlier (see page 22). Compared with people who had never smoked, this study found that smokers had an increased risk of dementia including Alzheimer's disease. Smoking was a strong risk factor for Alzheimer's disease in individuals without the ApoE 4 allele but had no effect in participants with this allele. The researchers stated that smoking was associated with a doubling of the risk of dementia and Alzheimer's disease.[1]

Another piece of research, which analysed prospective data from 21,123 people who participated in a survey between 1978 and 1985, looked at the association between midlife smoking and risk of dementia (Alzheimer's disease and vascular dementia).[2] This study showed that compared with non-smokers, those smoking more than two packs a day had a higher risk of dementia – a greater than 100% increase in risk. This increased risk was observed in those smoking more than two packs of cigarettes daily compared with those who did not smoke at all. However, for those who had given up smoking and for those smoking less than half a pack a day, no increased risk was noted. Significantly this study particularly concentrated on smoking in mid-life leading to dementia later in life.[2]

Contrast the above two papers with a study published in 2000 of 34,439 male British doctors who had been followed up since 1951. This study compared those who had continued to smoke with those who had either never smoked or counted themselves as ex-smokers. (Large numbers of doctors gave up smoking when the evidence that smoking was a major cause of premature death became clear.) Most of the ex-smokers had given up smoking up to more than 30 years before this study and so they were considered together with those who had never smoked. Interestingly this study concluded: 'Contrary to previous suggestions persistent smoking does not substantially reduce the age specific onset rate of Alzheimer's disease (AD) or of dementia in general. If anything, it might increase rather than decrease the rate, but any net effect on severe dementia cannot be large in either direction.'[3] In other words, smoking did not appear to make the onset of dementia arrive earlier. Indeed, the writers of this paper felt that any effect of smoking on the risk of dementia was negligible.[3]

The research specific to dementia then, is not necessarily conclusive. However, as has been pointed out in previous chapters, there are other physical diseases and events that may well predispose towards dementia. Smoking is known to increase the possibility of being affected by a stroke or of developing other vascular diseases, both of which are risk factors for dementia. A paper published in 2005 looked at the aggregate risk of various factors in connection with dementia. In this piece of research, 1138 people without dementia were followed up for 5.5 years and the researchers found that four risk factors – diabetes, hypertension, heart disease and current smoking – were associated with a higher risk of AD.[4] The risk of AD increased with the number of risk factors. Diabetes and current smoking were the strongest risk factors in isolation or in clusters, but hypertension and heart disease were also related to a higher risk of AD when clustered with diabetes, smoking or each other.

If you are keen to avoid the possibility of developing dementia it seems clear that avoiding or giving up a smoking habit is a wise move.

This brings us to another lifestyle habit which is constantly in the health news with often conflicting research results – drinking alcohol.

Alcohol

Before considering research into alcohol intake and dementia it is necessary to refer to one brain disorder which is usually (but not always) associated with heavy drinking and which is sometimes referred to – not totally correctly – as a form of dementia: Wernicke-Korsakoff syndrome. Wernicke's encephalopathy usually develops suddenly. It is due to a lack of thiamine (also known as vitamin B1). People who drink excessive amounts of alcohol are often thiamine deficient because of poor eating habits and because alcohol can interfere with the body's ability to convert thiamine into the active form of the vitamin. There are three main symptoms: involuntary, jerky eye movements or paralysis of muscles moving the eyes; poor balance, staggering gait or inability to walk; and drowsiness and confusion. If treated in time, by injections of thiamine, the symptoms are usually reversed in a few hours. However, if Wernicke's is left untreated, or is not treated in time, brain damage may result and Korsakoff's syndrome may develop. This results in short-term memory loss, changes in personality and attempts by the sufferer to make things up to fill the inevitable memory gaps.

Treatment for Korsakoff's syndrome consists of complete abstention from alcohol and injections of thiamine. Generally, someone who has developed this syndrome does not make a complete recovery but this treatment will prevent a deterioration of the condition. Sometimes this condition can result from poor nutrition without alcohol intake but this is rare in the western world.

The evidence for alcohol intake as a risk factor for the development of dementia itself is, if anything, even more confusing than the evidence concerning a smoking habit.

Research conducted as part of the Rotterdam Study (mentioned in Chapter 2) published in the *Lancet* in 2002 looked at the drinking habits of 7983 people aged 55 years and older.[5] This study concluded that compared to no alcohol consumption, light to moderate alcohol consumption was associated with a reduced risk of dementia in older adults. No variation in the protective value of any particular type of drink was noted. Light to moderate drinking was defined as one to three drinks per day.

One noted limitation of this study was the fact that levels of alcohol consumption were self-reported. There is a general belief within the medical profession that people under-report both the amount they smoke and the amount they drink. The researchers in this study suggested that the beneficial effects of low to moderate alcohol consumption might be because of a reduction in cardiovascular risk factors or it might be a direct effect on cognition of the release of acetylcholine in the part of the brain called the hippocampus. Acetylcholine is a neurotransmitter that is known to facilitate learning and memory. It is thought that a low concentration of alcohol stimulates the release of acetylcholine whereas higher concentrations inhibit this. Such an effect would suggest that heavy drinking increases the risk of dementia.

A review of research into connections between alcohol

intake and dementia by Luc Letenneur of the Université Victor Segalen in Bordeaux published in 2004 included reference to the above study and also to a well-known study conducted in France by researchers (including the author of this review) which specifically looked at wine consumption and risk of dementia. The people studied were visited at home by a psychologist and several characteristics were recorded, including wine consumption. In this study, moderate drinking was defined as three to four glasses of wine per day. A first analysis showed that moderate wine consumption was associated with a lower risk of incident dementia three years after the initial visit. When considering AD, mild drinkers and moderate drinkers had a significant decrease in risk.[6]

Another analysis confirmed these results after adjustment for many other potential confounding factors. This French study concluded that moderate drinking of alcohol was associated with a reduced risk of dementia.[7] The review also considered several similar studies conducted in parts of Europe and pointed out that the benefits of moderate alcohol intake seemed to be confined to men over the age of 40 and women over the age of 50. In younger people the consequences of alcohol consumption were more negative due to accidents and diseases directly linked to alcohol. This review suggested that the elderly should not be discouraged from drinking alcohol but concluded that it would be premature 'to advise people who did not drink to start drinking' in order to avoid developing dementia.[7]

More recently (2012), two studies were presented at the Alzheimer's Association International Conference in Vancouver. These studies found that moderate alcohol consumption later in life, heavier alcohol consumption earlier in life and binge drinking later in life increased the risk of declining cognitive performance.

The first study, by Tina Hoang and colleagues of NCIRE/ the Veterans' Health Research Institute, San Francisco and the

University of California, San Francisco and published in 2014, was conducted only on women. It followed more than 1300 women aged 65 and over for a period of 20 years. The results showed that women who had drunk greater amounts in the past and subsequently reduced their drinking had a 30% increased risk of cognitive performance decline. Participants who drank moderately (defined as 7-14 drinks per week) in the later phases of the study were approximately 60% more likely to develop cognitive impairment and women who changed from being non-drinkers to drinkers over the course of the study increased their risk of developing cognitive impairment by 200%. The researchers concluded that alcohol intake in later life might not be beneficial in older women.[8] Compare this with the study above suggesting that moderate alcohol intake seemed to benefit women over the age of 50.

The second study analysed data from 5075 US adults aged 65 and older over eight years. Cognitive function and memory were assessed using telephone interviews, and results showed that those who reported binge drinking (four or more drinks in one sitting) twice a month were more than twice as likely to experience a higher level of cognitive decline.[9] This study, of course, had the same limitations as the Rotterdam study in that the amount of drink consumed and the incidence of binge drinking were self-reported.

A 23-year follow-up study quoted in the *Lancet* report on dementia, 2020 (see Introduction), concluded that the dementia risk was increased in those who abstained from drinking alcohol in midlife and also (confusingly) in those who consumed more than 14 units of alcohol each week.[10] The *Lancet* report lists a reduction in alcohol consumption as one of the modifiable risk factors for dementia, but not all research backs this as we've seen.

Whatever might be concluded from the state of current research about the possibilities of alcohol consumption being a risk factor for the development of dementia in later life, we do know that alcohol consumption has a bad effect on someone who has dementia. This is obvious really. Even those of us who have no cognitive impairment have more difficulty in solving problems, carrying out complex tasks and driving a vehicle after consuming alcohol. If the brain is already under stress and cognitive performance is impaired, it would hardly seem sensible to administer a substance likely to make things worse! However, it is worth bearing in mind the advice given in Chapter 12 on what to do after a diagnosis. In general, people are happier and keep their quality of life longer if they continue to enjoy leisure pursuits which they took part in before the diagnosis. If you or the person you are caring for enjoyed a gin and tonic before dinner or a pint once a week, there is probably no harm in continuing this if your doctor agrees. However, bear in mind that memory problems may mean that someone with dementia forgets that they have had a drink so that one drink may become one drink after another without supervision!

Body weight

Body weight is another health area where dementia and other ill-health risks overlap. Most people acknowledge that they understand that being obese is a health risk. NHS UK suggests that obesity is linked to many areas of ill-health including type 2 diabetes, heart disease and arthritis. But some of the research concerning the connection between being overweight (rather than obese) and dementia has been equivocal.

Emiliano Albanese and colleagues conducted a meta-analysis (review of all the relevant published research) of much of the conflicting epidemiologic evidence on the association between midlife body mass index (BMI) and dementia and the results were published in 2017. They looked at 19 studies on 589,649 participants who were followed up for up to 42 years. This review concluded that midlife (age 35 to 65 years) obesity (but not overweight), was associated with dementia in late life.[11] This is a very interesting conclusion because the majority of people worried about their weight might not be considered to be obese but merely a few pounds overweight.

However, another study, investigating whether weight loss helped to improve cognition, found that '(intentional) weight loss was associated with a significant improvement in attention and memory' and that weight loss in both obese and overweight people was associated with improvements in performance across various cognitive domains (attention, memory, understanding, etc).[12]

Whether it affects your risk of dementia or not, obesity is bad for your heart health and most advice suggests keeping weight within acceptable parameters is a good policy.

Sleep

The importance of sleep patterns in avoiding dementia is another area which has been highlighted recently. It is generally accepted that poor sleeping patterns mean that we do not function as well in our daily life, as anyone who has suffered a 'broken night' can testify, but new evidence seems to indicate that regular chronic insomnia and poor sleeping patterns may increase the risk of later developing dementia.

It is not yet possible to confirm that bad sleep patterns (including not sleeping enough each night) actually increase the risk of dementia. However, there are plenty of reasons why a good night's sleep might be good for brain health. And there has been growing evidence to suggest sleep patterns before dementia onset may contribute to the disease. Insufficient time spent sleeping is linked to dementia risk in adults aged 65 and older.

A study led by Dr Séverine Sabia of Inserm and University College London examined how sleep patterns might affect the onset of dementia decades later. They looked at data from nearly

8000 individuals in Britain starting at age 50 and analysis of the data showed that people in mid-life (defined as people in their 50s and 60s) who were getting six hours or fewer of sleep were at greater risk of developing dementia later. Compared to those getting about seven hours sleep (which was considered 'normal'), those people sleeping less than six hours were 30% more likely to be diagnosed with dementia.[13] The researchers had taken into account other factors known to influence sleep patterns or dementia risk, such as physical exercise, body mass index and medical conditions like diabetes and heart disease.

The findings suggest that short sleep duration during midlife could increase the risk of developing dementia later in life. More research is needed to confirm this connection and understand the underlying reasons.

A small study which received a lot of media coverage has suggested that losing just one night of sleep led to an increase in beta-amyloid.[14] Beta-amyloid is a metabolic waste product that's found in the fluid between brain cells (neurones); it is cleared from the brain during sleep. This is part of the cleansing cycle which goes on in the body whilst we are asleep. In Alzheimer's disease, it has been found that beta-amyloid clumps together to form amyloid 'plaques', which cause problems with communication between neurones. The most recent research has indicated that the amyloid plaques are not a cause of dementia and studies that have involved drugs which reduce beta-amyloid plaques in the brain have now shown that clearing the plaques does not improve cognition. Nevertheless, a build-up of beta-amyloid is linked to impaired brain function.

Spouse/partner with dementia

Whilst not exactly a lifestyle choice, this chapter seems an appropriate place to mention an interesting and unusual piece of research. In 2010 Maria Norton and colleagues published a paper in the *Journal of the American Geriatric Society* which investigated whether spouses of people with dementia were at an increased risk of developing dementia themselves. The high level of stress experienced by spouse caregivers is well known and it is equally well known that stress has an effect on cognitive function. However, this research specifically investigated the risk to the spouse caregiver of later developing dementia.

It was found that spouses of those with dementia had a 600% greater risk of developing dementia than spouses of people without dementia. The authors reported a 'clear increased risk of incident dementia among older adults whose spouses have dementia'.[15]

This seems like quite a frightening finding and might make some people question the accepted conception that you cannot 'catch' dementia from someone who has it. However, as the authors pointed out, there might be several explanations for the finding of a greater risk in spouses. As far as possible the researchers themselves tried to adjust for socioeconomic status, and for any environmental factors such as a healthy or less healthy lifestyle shared by both spouses. However, it is possible that a shared lifestyle at least partially explained the findings. There are likely to be similarities in terms of diet, exercise pattern and personality type which increase the risk of dementia for both partners. Dementia in one partner leads to social isolation for both and social isolation is a major risk factor, as we have seen. Caregivers are also more likely to be depressed and to have less time to exercise or follow a hobby or interest of their own and these are potential risk factors for dementia (see Chapter 6 on mental health).

The authors were also careful to make the point that while the overall risk for dementia among married individuals whose spouse had dementia was high, many spouses were not affected.

Early menopause

The link between early menopause and dementia was not evident when I wrote the first edition of this book. However, a study published in 2022 suggested that people who entered menopause early (this was defined as before the age of 45) might be at a higher risk for having dementia later in life. The study was presented in March 2022 at a conference of the American Heart Association. It examined health data from 153,291 women in the United Kingdom.[16] It found that women who experienced an early menopause were 30% more likely to be diagnosed with dementia before age 65 than those whose periods ceased at 50. Note, however, that this is an 'observational study' which could not identify a specific reason for the link between earlier menopause and possible higher dementia risk. One theory is that reduced oestrogen levels at a younger age may be a factor but more study is needed to determine this. It is worth noting that the study didn't include information on family history of dementia.

Conclusion

Scientific research is divided on how personality traits affect the likelihood of dementia development. The evidence concerning lifestyle choices and some of the miscellaneous factors outlined above is also not completely clear-cut. However, the research and evidence reproduced in this chapter highlight some of the lifestyle choices which seem to increase the risk of developing dementia. In Part III of this book we will be looking at what steps we as individuals can take to decrease our risk factors.

Chapter 4

Drugs and dementia

By Dr Jerry Thompson, GP

- Drugs used for Alzheimer's disease:
  - The latest drug
  - Why there are no new drug discoveries
- Is there another way? The Bredesen Program
- Could your medication be part of the problem?
  - The two monsters: statins and PPIs
  - Other drugs linked with dementia
- Other substances linked with dementia

As you're reading this book, I assume that you, the reader, have an interest in dementia. Perhaps it is because you have a family member affected? Or perhaps you have early signs of dementia yourself? Either way, it would help to have an understanding of which drugs are used in Alzheimer's disease (or any other form of dementia) and how other commonly-used drugs could impact on this disease.

Alzheimer's disease is the commonest form of dementia and most of the research is on Alzheimer's so I think it's reasonable to assume that what follows that applies to Alzheimer's disease applies to dementia as a whole, although only time will tell.

The first question, is what drugs are available? The second is, what are the real benefits and the downsides of these drugs? Then we need to think about whether any other drugs you are using could be making matters worse. Let me start with an example.

Case history

Several years ago, I saw a patient who was in his eighties. Let's call him Jim. His wife brought him in suspecting that he was developing dementia. Jim was virtually monosyllabic, and I couldn't get much sense out of him. I asked the usual questions, which were largely answered by his wife. She thought he could have dementia. I felt her suspicions were likely to be correct and suggested we did some screening tests and then refer him to the memory clinic.

However, I noticed something else about Jim. His blood tests revealed his cholesterol was abnormally low; it was about 3.0 mmol/l. The reason was easy to find. It was due to the statin drug he was taking. This combination of low cholesterol and possible dementia set alarm bells ringing in my mind.

I was aware of a key study which followed nearly 2000 people. It demonstrated that the lower a person's cholesterol, the worse their brain performance. (In this study, the researchers had measured verbal fluency, attention, concentration and abstract reasoning.)[1] They found mental function drops progressively once cholesterol goes below 4.6 mmol/l. This research worried me because I had been seeing more and more people with very low cholesterol levels, all since statins had started being widely prescribed.

While we were investigating Jim, I suggested he stop the statins and see how he got on without them. I saw him about six weeks later and hardly recognised him as the same person. He was talking freely and confirmed that his mental fog had lifted. I was only too pleased for him.

At this point an uncomfortable thought came to my mind. I wondered how many other people there were out there, like Jim, who had sunk into a drug-induced oblivion. I suspected that this completely correctable loss of brain function was only too common and often missed.

My experience is that most doctors overestimate the dangers of high cholesterol but underestimate the dangers of low cholesterol. And low cholesterol is not just linked with mental decline; it is linked with increased mortality.

Drugs used for Alzheimer's disease

With any illness, it's crucial to know what treatment is available and how good it is. Even if it turns out that there are no good drugs at present, you would want to know if there could be a cure coming up in the near future. After all, there are stories in the media almost every day about some research which could cure this or that disease, often with the suggestion that a new drug is just round the corner. In reality, genuine new drug discoveries are rare and often not what they are cracked up to be.

So let's look at the facts. There are presently four drugs licensed in the UK for Alzheimer's disease. They are all old, in fact, very old. No new drugs have become available since 2002. Another drug has recently been licensed in the USA but not in the UK or Europe, and further drugs of a similar type may be marketed soon. We will look at these later (see page 61). One drug made it to the market but was withdrawn due to severe liver toxicity (Tacrine). None of the drugs presently available alters the course of the disease. There are still over 100 drugs in the pipeline, but these are thought to be newer variations of the drugs currently available.

Initially things were different. Pharmaceutical companies recognised that dementia was a potentially huge market and they invested heavily (having spent an estimated $42 billion in 25 years). They knew that people with Alzheimer's disease had very low levels of the neurotransmitter acetylcholine, which is reduced by as much as 90% in dementia. Acetylcholine is essential for nerve transmission and important for memory. The race was on to find a drug that could increase acetylcholine and thereby potentially cure dementia.

They developed drugs called cholinesterase inhibitors (cholinesterase breaks down acetylcholine), which were expected to increase the levels of acetylcholine. Unfortunately, these drugs did not live up to expectations and were far from a cure for dementia.

But what of the drugs that made it to market? Three are cholinesterase inhibitors – namely, donepizil (trade names include Aricept), rivastigmine (trade names include Exelon) and galantamine (trade names include Reminyl, Acumar and Galasya). The odd man out is memantine (trade names include Ebixa, Maruxa and Nemdatine). This is a NMDA receptor blocker. This inhibits glutamine, not cholinesterase. However, in reality it acts very much like a cholinesterase inhibitor.

All these drugs have been disappointing: all have been found to give only minor benefits. None slows the progression of the disease. Although they successfully block cholinesterase, the brain compensates by producing more of the enzyme. This creates a further problem: if the patient stops the drug, symptoms worsen. Another issue is adverse effects. Cholinesterase inhibitors can cause a wide range of these: nausea, vomiting, diarrhoea, insomnia, bizarre dreams, cramps and fatigue, whilst memantine can cause dizziness, drowsiness, agitation and hallucinations. A problem for carers is that it is not easy to distinguish drug side-effects from a flare-up of the dementia.

There is, however, a postscript to the story of dementia

drugs. A study was published in November 2018 that reviewed 10 studies involving a total of 2714 patients who received cholinesterase inhibitors or memantine. After pooling the data, the study's authors found a significantly greater annual decline in mental function in patients on these drugs compared with those on no drugs. Those on both drugs did the worst.[2]

The latest drugs

The first new drug in 20 years to be approved in the USA (but not in Europe and the UK) was aducanumab (Aduhelm). For many years it was thought Alzheimer's disease was caused by a build-up of beta-amyloid plaque in the brain. However, there have been 30 unsuccessful trials of drugs that lower amyloid, but these have made no difference to mental function. Some drugs did successfully reduce amyloid but also worsened mental function.

Aducanumab was approved for early-stage dementia by the FDA (Food and Drug Administration) in the USA in June 2021. This approval was heavily criticised by neurologists and scientists. After it was approved by the FDA, three of the FDA experts resigned within days.

Aducanumab targets amyloid. It is given by infusion (not easy in a dementia patient) and has been noted to cause brain oedema (that is, swelling – not easy to diagnose in a dementia patient) in as many as 35% of cases, and to cause micro-haemorrhages in 19%. This means regular MRI scans need to be done on all patients taking it (again, not always easy or even possible to do in dementia patients). The drug costs approximately £43,000 a year. Two trials showed it was ineffective and one showed some benefit.

You may wonder why it hasn't been approved in the UK or Europe? The controversy surrounding this drug was that it was approved for its benefit on what is called a 'surrogate endpoint'. In this case it was approved because it removed amyloid, not

61

because it gave any clinical benefit. Given what we know about amyloid and unsuccessful results of previous trials of drugs that targeted amyloid, this was hardly a surprise. So this was indeed a bizarre decision.

The European Medicines Agency (EMA) refused to give it a licence in December 2021.

While this controversy has been going on, another drug has been developed, called lecanemab. It is similar to aducanumab in that it targets amyloid, although a different type of amyloid. It is also given by infusion (every two weeks). Like aducanumab it can cause brain oedema and bleeding (this occurred in 23% in the trial described next).

A trial of lecanemab in 1795 people caused excitement as it was found to reduce cognitive decline by 27% over 18 months. The reality was less striking: the difference between scores on patients taking the drug and those taking placebo was 0.45 on an 18-point clinical scale of dementia. In other words, this change was small and probably barely noticeable. It might have benefits, but it was far from a cure for dementia. Despite this, the drug has been fast-tracked for approval.

Since then a third drug, donanemab, has made the headlines. This also targets amyloid. Like lecanemab, it showed a small benefit, reducing decline in Alzheimer's dementia by 10 points on a 144 point scale (compared to 13 with placebo) over 18 months. However, a quarter of patients developed brain oedema or bleeding whilst on the drug. Infusion reactions occurred in 9% and three people died whilst taking donanemab (one on placebo). As you can see, it is far from clear if the benefits of the drug outweigh the risks.

Few people have heard of the fourth drug of this class, solanezumab. This works in the same way and again successfully stops the amyloid burden increasing in preclinical Alzheimer's disease. However, this drug did not help with cognitive function.

I've covered dementia drugs in some detail here. As you can

see, there is no current treatment which gives any meaningful benefit and some could even be making things worse. Sadly, there is little prospect of a new pharmaceutical wonder drug around the corner any time soon.

Why are there no new drug discoveries?

You might be surprised about the lack of success, given the huge sums of money thrown at dementia. In fact, we don't need to look far to understand why.

Although mainstream medicine has been highly effective in curing acute conditions (infections, fractures, surgical emergencies), it has had virtually zero success in treating chronic diseases. Even with cancer, it is usually early surgery rather than drugs that leads to cure. Apart from a few rare conditions, we can say that virtually no chronic disease has been cured. So perhaps we shouldn't be too surprised that no cure has been found for dementia.

The strategy of pharmaceutical companies has typically been to create drugs which block pathways in the body – beta-blockers, antihistamines, antidepressants and, in this case, cholinesterase inhibitors. This is good for symptom relief but not useful when it comes to curing an illness.

A newer development is to use monoclonal antibodies to target certain body structures. These drugs usually end in 'mab', short for monoclonal antibody, and include aducanumab, lecanemab and donanemab, which we have previously met and which target amyloid. Some of these monoclonal antibodies have had major benefits, in terms of relieving symptoms when used in other diseases, but none has led to a cure. They are extremely expensive. They also alter immunity, predisposing those who take them to serious infections.

Is there another way?

There is another way, but this is an untold story about dementia. Many people do recover from chronic diseases and they are doing so increasingly, but these cures require a different way of thinking. This involves looking for the causes of the disease and then increasing the elements supporting the body (such good nutrition, exercise and sleep) and removing damaging factors (such as stress, toxicity, allergy and inflammation). Eventually the body reaches a tipping point where recovery occurs.

Dr Dale Bredesen had spent much of his life researching the brain and established his own laboratory at UCLA (University of California, Los Angeles) in 1989. During this time, he had a personal experience of this other type of medicine. His teenage daughter developed lupus, an autoimmune disease. He saw two top specialists in the field of lupus. Neither seemed interested in the underlying cause and all they could offer his daughter was steroids when the illness flared up. This is typical of mainstream medicine for chronic disease: good for accurate diagnosis but short on ideas when it comes to treatment.

Bredesen knew he had to think outside the box and turned to a doctor in integrative medicine, even though this doctor had no specific expertise in lupus. This doctor changed her diet, used supplements and balanced her hormones. It was a personalised approach. His daughter made a full recovery and has continued in good health for the last 10 years. The importance of this was not lost on Bredesen when he started researching dementia.

Bredesen went on to make what might be one of the greatest discoveries in dementia. He found what he considered to be the underlying mechanism. To his surprise, he found Alzheimer's disease could arise due to a protective mechanism: if the brain doesn't have enough brain-nourishing substances available (notably brain-derived neurotrophic factor (BNF) and netrin-1) or has an excess of toxic substances to deal with (including amyloid and biotoxins), it has to shut down some parts of itself to preserve function in the more essential areas.

It all hinges on a molecule that sits on the nerve receptor called APP (amyloid precursor protein) and the way it breaks down. If all is well, APP breaks down into two nerve-nourishing substances and the brain functions normally. If the brain is faced with deficiencies or toxic substances and has to use this protective mechanism, it instead produces four nerve-damaging substances.

He also found that, by controlling the various factors that influence APP, it was possible to tip the balance away from nerve destruction and towards nerve creation.

Bredesen discovered 36 key factors[3] that influence the breakdown of APP. He developed the Bredesen protocol (called ReCODE) and applied to have it tested (like a drug). This was turned down. He was told it was too complex, although ironically it is this very complexity that explains why no present drug treatment has been successful to this day. (For more information see Bredesen's book, *The End of Alzheimer's.*[3])

Despite this negative response, he went on to do clinical trials of his protocol. In 2014 he published a study of 100 patients from clinics in the USA and Australia who went through the protocol. Nine out of 10 patients with early Alzheimer's disease showed reversal of mental decline.[4] This had never been achieved before. These results have been replicated in two further peer-reviewed studies.[4, 5, 6]

The ReCODE has now been successfully used in over 1000 patients in seven countries. Virtually all patients with mild Alzheimer's disease improve. In moderate disease, 50% improve. Only a minority improve with advanced Alzheimer's disease.

He has identified three different subtypes of dementia:

1. Inflammatory (often related to the ApoE4 gene – see page 94), this subgroup typically responds well to the protocol.
2. Atrophic (also related to the ApoE4 gene), responds well

but more slowly. This type can also be associated with high levels of glucose, insulin or homocysteine.

3. Toxic, which is unrelated to the ApoE4 gene and is the hardest to treat. It can be caused by heavy metals, such as mercury and aluminium, and other toxic chemicals.

He has since added two further categories: vascular and traumatic.

The Bredesen program

The first step of the protocol involves looking at 35 'holes' (mechanisms).[7] Typically, he found 25 were low or suboptimal and needed correcting. This varies from patient to patient so, again, this method needs a personalised approach.

It typically takes six months for the pathological brain changes to reverse, and the condition can return within a few weeks of stopping the protocol. Consequently, perseverance with the protocol is essential. A good source of information on the Bredesen method is www.apollohealthco.com.

Why new ideas are slow to be accepted in medicine

So you might well ask why patients are treated with largely ineffective drugs when we have peer-reviewed published evidence of an effective treatment for dementia (at least in the early stages). Sadly, medicine has a long history of ignoring successful treatments if they involve a new way of thinking.

A classic example of this relates to Australian researchers, Barry Marshall and Robin Warren. They eventually received the Nobel Prize in Medicine and Physiology for discovering that the bacterium *Helicobacter pylori* was a major cause of peptic ulcers. However, the medical profession was so wedded to the idea that bacteria could not live in the stomach that Barry Marshall had to resort to the drastic step of infecting himself to get his point across.

Another major reason why the Bredesen protocol hasn't come to light is that the cure involves using natural substances which cannot be patented. This means there is no money to be made by pharmaceutical companies and hence there is no money to support research. Again this is a common story in the history of medicine and helps to explain why progress in medicine has often been so painfully slow.

Another issue is that the treatment is complex because of the need to look at all the possible underlying causes and correct them individually. At the moment there aren't many practitioners who are familiar with the ReCODE protocol.

Could your medication be part of the problem?

There's another aspect to drugs and Alzheimer's disease as illustrated by Jim's story at the start of this chapter. Could your present medication be part of the problem? I'm going to start with what I will call the two 'pharmaceutical monsters'. I'm calling them that because they are so widely prescribed that it seems almost everybody over a certain age is taking them. Then I'll look through some other drugs that can make dementia worse.

The two monsters: Statins and PPIs

Statins

According to some estimates, about 11 million people in the UK are taking statins. However, are these drugs linked with memory problems?

The answer is yes. One condition known to be caused by statins is transient global amnesia. Here a person suddenly loses their memory. They don't know where they are or how they got there. This can be terrifying. And yet they know who they are, can recognise familiar faces and can perform complex tasks. It can last hours to most of the day. There is even a book written by a former NASA doctor, who suffered from this himself after taking statins; the book is called *Lipitor, Thief of Memory*.[8] (Lipitor is the trade name for atorvastatin).

Recognised adverse effects of statins include forgetfulness, memory loss and confusion. They are also thought to cause a condition caused 'reversible cognitive decline'. This is probably what happened to Jim, as discussed above. Clearly, memory issues are a major concern with statins.

Statins are also linked with a number of other neurological conditions. They increase the risk of peripheral neuropathy by four to 16-fold, but 26-fold if statins have been taken for over two years.[9] They also are associated with a nine to 20-fold higher risk of motor neurone disease.[10]

Paradoxically, statins have been shown to reduce the risk of dementia and cognitive impairment in some people, although this benefit has not shown up in controlled trials.

But what we really need to know is what happens to the memory of individual patients taking statins. To do this, you need to take them off statins and then reintroduce the drugs. This is exactly what was done in a study of 18 patients with mild dementia. These patients were taken off statins for six weeks and then put back on them for six weeks. The results were clear cut. When taken off the statin, their MMSE score (mini-mental state examination) went up by 2 points on average and other measures of mental function improved, including verbal memory. To put this in perspective, an increase of 4 points in MMSE would have taken them into the normal (non-dementia) range. The MMSE scores declined again on going back on statins. This is a very practical study, demonstrating the negative effect of these drugs on memory.[11]

Where does that leave us? I think we can explain this conundrum by noting the different effects of statins. They reduce cholesterol and this is known to impair mental function. Cholesterol is essential for the brain and 20% of all our cholesterol is in our brain. Cholesterol is severely deficient in diseased brains. Our ability to grow new nerve synapses depends on how much cholesterol is available. However, statins have other effects apart from reducing cholesterol. These include an anti-inflammatory effect, consequently having a slight beneficial effect on arterial disease. Which effect will predominate in one person is anyone's guess.

My major concern, as mentioned in the case of Jim previously, is that so-called reversible cognitive decline may not be picked up as a drug side-effect and could be put down to old age. If the patient is not taken off the statin, it will likely become a permanent cognitive decline with devastating long-term consequences. For these reasons I think statins need to be used with extreme caution.

In my opinion, statins should never be prescribed where there is deteriorating mental function or dementia. Sometimes they are given in vascular dementia and there is a certain logic to this. Despite this, studies on individuals with vascular disease given statins late in life have found they do not protect against dementia so there is no justification for using them.[12]

Proton pump inhibitors (PPIs)

PPIs block stomach acid. The most prescribed PPIs are omeprazole and lansoprazole. There are a number of reasons to be concerned about these drugs. They increase mortality by 25% in some studies[13] and increase cardiac mortality by 16-18%. In addition, they reduce the absorption of many vitamins and minerals crucial for brain function, notably B12. Raised homocysteine is a known risk factor for dementia and B12 deficiency is one cause of this.

But have studies shown an increase in dementia in people taking PPIs? Some have. A review of six studies with a total of

166,146 participants followed up for five years showed a 29% increase in dementia (39% in those over 65).[14] Another study of 73,679 patients over 75 taken from German Insurance data showed a 44% increase in dementia compared with those not using PPIs.[15] Another smaller German study of 3327 patients aged over 75 showed a 38% increase in dementia. However, it is true that not all studies of PPIs have shown an increase in dementia.

Studies on mice also support the view that PPIs increase dementia. Mice given PPIs developed increases in amyloid in their brains similar to that seen in humans with dementia.

Unlike statins, PPIs are difficult to stop. Rebound stomach acidity is a predictable and troublesome problem when attempting to come off these drugs. Usually coming off PPIs has to be done slowly and carefully.

On balance I think PPIs are likely to aggravate dementia and I would advise anyone at risk to avoid these. They are a hugely overprescribed drug, given the fact they are known to increase the risk of premature death, and should be used only for short periods and even then with great care.

Other pharmaceutical drugs linked with dementia

Remember acetylcholine, the substance needed for nerve transmission? As you know, it is very low in people with dementia. So you won't be surprised to hear that drugs which reduce acetylcholine can make dementia more likely. These are the anti-cholinergic drugs and there are a large number of them. Some have much stronger effects than others. It is thought 10% of people take drugs with anti-cholinergic properties.

In a study of 40,770 people aged 65-99 published in the *British Medical Journal*, researchers looked at the records of people who had taken these drugs from 2000 to 2015 and compared them with those of 283,933 controls. What they found was that three groups of anti-cholinergic drugs increased the risk of dementia. As expected, the strongest anti-cholinergic drugs had the biggest effects.[16]

The biggest increase in risk of dementia (45%) came from an anti-Parkinson's drug called procyclidine. Fortunately, this is rarely used these days. The second biggest risk (it caused a 23% higher risk of dementia) came from drugs used for the bladder (oxybutynin and tolterodine). The final group were antidepressants (which increased the risk by 13%). These included amitriptyline, dosulepin and paroxetine. The longer people had been on the drugs, the worse the outcome.

An unexpected finding was that, even when people had taken the drugs 15 to 20 years previously, the risk of dementia remained, suggesting long-term harm.[15] Other research in Germany and France has confirmed these findings.

Other drugs like antihistamines have a milder anti-cholinergic effect but another study showed prolonged use of first-generation antihistamines can cause dementia. A clue to whether a drug has a significant anti-cholinergic effect is if it gives you a dry mouth. For instance, the highest users of diphenhydramine (Benzadryl) had a 54% increased risk of dementia[16, 17] in one study. Another first-generation antihistamine is chlorphenamine (Piriton).

A range of other drugs has been found to increase the risk of dementia, including beta-blockers, benzodiazepines, warfarin, opioid painkillers and anticonvulsants.

Other substances linked with dementia

It's not just drugs that put us at risk. What we eat and drink makes a difference. Researchers looking at 1484 people over the age of 60 found a nearly 300% increase in dementia in those who took one or two diet drinks daily.[18] Most diet drinks contain aspartame which is converted in the body to formaldehyde, which is a potent neurotoxin.

Conclusion

So what should we do if faced with signs of dementia in either ourselves or someone close? One of the first steps is to consider whether any medication being taken is contributing to the symptoms. Coming off a drug is likely to require the support of your doctor to ensure there are no withdrawal problems and that the health problem for which the drug was prescribed can be managed in another way.

Currently there are no drugs available that can make a real difference to the treatment of dementia, and nothing promising is in the pipeline.

Chapter 5

Nutrition and dodging dementia

- Our bodies need a balance of protein, fat and carbohydrate but what that balance should be continues to be debated.
- Fats and cholesterol are essential for the brain to function.
- Eating oily fish is considered to be protective against dementia.
- Some research suggests that cutting calories from carbohydrates may help prevent dementia.
- Some vitamins and supplements may help but evidence for this is somewhat controversial.
- Despite all the controversy, it is generally agreed that if you have a dementia diagnosis, you should eat a 'nutrient-rich' diet.

'You are what you eat' the saying goes and indeed much government health advice these days centres around what we eat, how much we eat and how we 'should' be eating. Diet-related ill-health is now believed to be the leading cause of chronic disease around the world.[1] It may appear surprising then that comparatively little research has been done on the effects of diet on dementia and the risks of dementia.

Just as our bones and muscles need to be fed properly in order to function correctly, so too do our brains need to be fed in order to work at the optimal level. The physical body and the brain are both composed of body cells. The food principally used by the brain for fuel is glucose (see next).

Balancing protein, fats and carbohydrates

Many of us were taught at school about the body's basic dietary requirements for protein, fats and carbohydrates, the 'macro-nutrients' that provide energy and are used to build our body tissues.

Put simply, **proteins** are required for bodily growth and repair to tissues, as for example during recovery from injury. We need proteins every day to remain healthy as our bodies cannot store them in any quantity. Proteins are made up of chains of amino acids. There are eight amino acids which are essential to the body and have to be obtained from food as our bodies cannot make them. Meat, fish, eggs and dairy-produce all contain the eight essential amino acids in the proportions needed by the body. Other foods such as nuts, legumes (peas, beans and lentils) and seeds contain some of the essential amino acids and can be eaten in combination to provide the body with the right amino acid mixture. Strict vegans have to be careful to eat both adequate amounts and an adequate variety of protein-containing foods to ensure a sufficient supply of essential amino acids.

Fats are essential structurally and are also a fuel that can be stored. They provide energy for the growth and maintenance of body tissues, are essential constituents of all cell membranes and help to maintain body temperature. They also provide fat-soluble vitamins. A sufficient amount of fat in our diet causes us to feel full and prevents us overeating. An excess of fat will cause us to feel sick. To supply the essential fatty acids needed for proper functioning of the brain we need to eat at least 15 grams of these each day. As well as the obvious fat on meat and in butter and cooking fats/oils, fat is found in oily fish, milk, cheese and condiments such as mayonnaise. Some foods such as nuts and seeds have quite a high fat content, although this may not be obvious. Do not be misled by the simple (and erroneous) statement commonly read in popular literature that 'eating fat makes you fat'. When fat is digested it is oxidised by the body to provide energy for tissue activity and for the maintenance of body temperature. Deposits of fat around the vital organs of the body hold these organs in position and protect them from damage.

Fat is particularly important in the structure of the brain and nervous tissue. We need a steady intake of fat for the brain to function properly. Fats make up 60% of the brain and the nerves that run every system in the body. The body needs two kinds of fat to manufacture healthy brain cells, hormones and prostaglandins, essential locally-acting chemical messengers in the body. These are omega-6 fats (linoleic acid) and omega-3 fats (alpha linolenic acid). These are often known as 'essential fatty acids' and more is written about them later in this chapter.

Then a word about cholesterol as this has had a very bad press. Cholesterol is a fatty substance known as a lipid and is *vital* for the normal functioning of the body. It is essential for normal bodily functioning and is the precursor to many hormones. It is mainly made by the liver but can also be found in some foods we eat. It is needed everywhere in the brain, as an antioxidant and to manufacture neurotransmitters. It is dangerous to have levels of cholesterol that are too low (see more about cholesterol in Chapter 8).

As with fats, **carbohydrates** also provide energy. Most people think of foods like bread and potatoes when they consider the word carbohydrates but it is important to remember that all sugars and starches are carbohydrates. This includes sucrose (table sugar) and fructose which is the sugar found in fruit. After absorption in the intestines, the products of carbohydrates (sugars) are processed by the liver and utilised to produce energy. Excess sugars are converted into fat. If insufficient carbohydrate is taken in the diet to produce the required glucose, then the body can convert protein into glucose in a process called 'gluco-neogenesis'. It is clear that the production of glucose is important for life. However, the body can also convert fat into ketones to produce energy – see the note on ketones below.

The healthy level of glucose in the blood is generally agreed to be between 4 and 5.6 mmol/l and the body regulates this with the hormone insulin, which diverts glucose into cells where it is needed for energy and surplus sugar into fat cells for storage. If high levels of glucose are absorbed quickly, large amounts of insulin will be produced and blood glucose levels may come crashing down as a result. This 'boom and bust' is not healthy. Equally, constantly high levels of insulin in response to ongoing snacking on high-carb foods such as crisps and sweets can lead to 'insulin resistance', the precursor of type 2 diabetes which is one of the biggest risk factors for dementia, as we saw on page 31.

In order to produce the desirable slow and sustained release of glucose into the bloodstream, the diet should not be too high in carbohydrates, and especially refined carbohydrates (white bread, white flour etc), which tend to produce the 'spike' in blood sugar levels mentioned. Every meal should contain protein and fat to satisfy your appetite but not necessarily carbohydrate.

Meals should be eaten at regular intervals. If they are properly balanced and eaten at regular intervals than additional snacks should not be necessary or even desired. This doesn't mean that you should not treat yourself to the occasional slice of cake with your afternoon tea. It means that if you actually *need* that slice of cake in order to last out until the next meal then either your diet is not properly balanced or your meals are too far apart from each other.

The body also requires a supply of vitamins, minerals and trace elements to function correctly. The most common advice is that if the diet is adequate in respect of protein, fats and carbohydrates then a sufficient supply of vitamins, minerals and trace elements will be taken in. However, this is not necessarily true and we need to consider the elements of the diet in more detail.

The controversy: What is a balanced diet?

Standard current dietary advice is based around what is considered to be 'good' for the health of our heart and cardiac system. Broadly the official advice is to base our diet around carbohydrates, to reduce our intake of fats, increase our intake of fruit and vegetables and to keep cholesterol levels low. Whilst this diet is popularly considered to be a 'healthy heart diet' for those in mid-life, some specific research shows that in adopting this way of eating we are no longer giving our brain the optimum diet. As explained above, in order to work properly the brain needs dietary fat, cholesterol and a *steady* supply of glucose.

What is becoming clear from research is that there is a definite link between excess dietary carbohydrates (particularly the sugar called fructose) along with a deficiency in dietary fats and cholesterol which may lead to the development of Alzheimer's disease.

One paper published in the *Journal of Neurochemistry* in 2008 pointed out that in trials a reduced carbohydrate intake prevented Alzheimer's disease-type amyloidosis (a condition where proteins are abnormally deposited in organs or tissues and cause harm). This paper mentioned the term 'metabolic syndrome', which is a term for a group of risk factors that occur together and are thought to increase the risk of coronary artery disease, stroke and type 2 diabetes. The suggestion is that this syndrome also increases the risk of Alzheimer's disease and the syndrome is linked to high calorie intake and diets high in sugar and refined flour. The authors recommended that those at risk of Alzheimer's disease eat whole and unrefined foods with natural fats, especially fish, nuts and seeds, olives and olive oil, and reduce the intake of foods that disrupt insulin and the blood sugar balance.[2]

A 2011 paper published in the *European Journal of Internal Medicine* pointed out that the cerebrospinal fluid in the brains of people with Alzheimer's disease was deficient in fats and cholesterol and suggested that Alzheimer's disease might be caused by a deficiency in the supply chain of cholesterol, fats and antioxidants to the brain.[3] This paper suggested that a diet high in high-glycaemic carbohydrates (carbs that are absorbed quickly and so spike blood sugar levels, especially fructose) and low in cholesterol and fats began the process that leads to neuronal failure. The authors proposed that dietary modifications resulting in fewer highly processed carbohydrates and more fats and cholesterol would be a protective measure against Alzheimer's disease.

We have seen that neurones are involved in the transmission of signals in the brain and throughout the nervous system. Astrocytes (also known as 'glia') are the cells that supply cholesterol, fats and glucose to the neurones. It is believed that excess exposure to glucose and to oxidising agents can lead to damage in the astrocytes. This, said the authors of the paper, will lead to defects in the transmission of neural signals.[3]

Cutting calories?

Some animal-based research has suggested that cutting calories overall may halt or even reverse the symptoms of Alzheimer's disease. Published in the *Journal of Alzheimer's Disease*, this study involved a team of researchers from the Mount Sinai School of Medicine in New York City maintaining a group of squirrel monkeys on either calorie-restricted or 'normal' diets throughout their lifespan. Compared with those on a 'normal' diet, the monkeys that were fed the reduced-calorie diet were less likely to have Alzheimer's disease-type changes in their brains.[4] The reduced-calorie diet was also associated with increased longevity of a protein known as SIRT1, which influences a variety of functions, including age-related diseases.

Some more recent research comparing the effects of following the MIND diet (a modified form of the Mediterranean diet – see Chapter 8) seems to bear out these results.[5]

The significance of this research is reflected in further studies around ketones (see below). However, when considering a reduced-calorie diet, it is also important to remember that many elderly people may be in a poor nutritional state due to increasing frailty, lack of exposure to sunlight and an inability to shop for food and prepare meals because of cognitive impairment or physical disability. If someone is already suffering from under-nutrition, it would be quite inappropriate to suggest a reduction in calories. Instead, action to enrich the diet should be taken in accordance with the suggestions given at the end of this chapter.

Research has already indicated a clear link between Alzheimer's disease and diabetes (see Chapter 2, page 31). A diet high in processed carbohydrates like bread, breakfast cereals and fruit juices, particularly if this diet is also low in fats, results in a rapid rise in blood glucose levels after meals. Over time it is believed that this may lead to insulin resistance (as described above) and diabetes.

One of the most interesting links between nutrition and the risk of dementia was the subject of a piece of research which showed a link between the nutritional status of mothers in pregnancy and the development of dementia in their children in later life. At the end of World War II a severe famine occurred in cities in the western part of the Netherlands. At one stage, rations were as low as 400 calories per day. This study found that in late middle life (age 56-59 years) people exposed to famine during the early stage of gestation performed worse than expected on selective attention tasks.[6]

Conclusion

Eating a well-balanced diet with sufficient levels of proteins, fats and carbohydrates will give a controlled release of glucose, ensure we have the nutrients we need to stay healthy and help to protect against dementia. Recent research indicates that not all current 'accepted' advice about low-fat, high-carbohydrate diets and restricting cholesterol should necessarily apply to older people wishing to protect themselves against dementia. It appears that simple dietary modification towards fewer highly processed carbohydrates and relatively more fats and cholesterol is likely to be a protective measure against Alzheimer's disease.

Essential fatty acids: Omega-6 and omega-3

Omega-6 and omega-3 fatty acids, as previously mentioned, are often known as 'essential' fatty acids because they must be obtained from our food – we can't make them for ourselves. There are three types of omega-3: alpha-linolenic acid (ALA) found in nuts and seeds, and eicosapentaenoic acid (EPA) and docosahexaenoic acid (DHA), both found in oily fish and grass-fed meat, and also in marine algae. ALA is thought to help reduce heart disease; EPA and DHA help maintain the tissues of the eye and brain. Our bodies can convert ALA to EPA and DHA if we have the right enzymes, so it is possible though more difficult to obtain all the omega-3 we need from plant sources.

Omega-6 fatty acids come in two forms: linoleic acid (LA) and arachidonic acid (AA). These are the prime structural components of brain cell membranes and are also an important part of the enzymes within cell membranes that allow the membranes to transport valuable nutrients in and out of the cells.

Omega-6 fatty acids are found in a wide variety of foods including plant/seed oils (notably evening primrose oil) as well as meat and animal products and it is believed that a shortage of this type of fat is rare in most Western diets. Of particular concern is processed omega-6 fats which, owing to high temperatures or the process of 'hydrogenation' that makes them solid at room temperature (as in 'spreads') can be transformed into trans fats that the body cannot use healthily. These need to be avoided.

Omega-3 is found generally in oily fish as well as in some oils, nuts and seeds. Most advice centres around the suggestion that we increase our intake of omega-3 in order to balance our intake of omega-6. However, the simple fact is that there is very little consensus among nutritionists about how much omega-3 and omega-6 oils are needed in total for optimum health and about the ideal ratio between the two, although it is believed that Western diets do not have a healthy balance.[7] While in theory a higher level of omega-3 fatty acids relative to omega 6 are better for our health, and many recommended diets (such as the Mediterranean Diet) give a ratio of 4 omega-6 to 1 omega-3 as ideal, this is not necessarily exactly supported by evidence.

As far as there is any consensus it seems to centre on the suggestion that for the good of the health of our hearts and our brains we should all be eating more oily fish. A research paper looking at fish consumption and cognitive function in people without dementia showed that 'there were significant positive associations between reported fish consumption and the CVLT (Californian Verbal Learning Test) scores' and concluded: 'We have demonstrated a positive association between reported fish consumption and cognitive function in a large sample of healthy older people in the UK.'[8]

The usual recommendation is two servings of oily fish per week. The word 'oily' seems to put many people off but in fact this term includes a number of different species which makes it easier to include these in the diet. Oily fish include mackerel, herring, salmon, whitebait, sardines, trout, pilchards, kippers, eels, fresh tuna, anchovies, swordfish and sprats. Tinned tuna is not included in this list because the canning process is thought to negate the omega-3 content. However, high-quality brands canned in water rather than oil can in fact contain significant amounts. You need to read the label. Vegetarians can get omega-3 from flaxseed, hempseed, nuts and (if eaten) eggs.

Given such a comprehensive list, you may begin to think that increasing our omega-3 intake not so difficult.

Ketones

An interesting piece of information and anecdotal evidence has come from the USA. A Florida doctor, Dr Mary Newport, who was married to a man who had dementia, read about coconut oil and began dosing her husband with this. She claimed that he showed a remarkable improvement on this regime and submitted some of his test results to bear out his recovery in her book.[9] The improvements to her husband's cognition were not all maintained and this type of initial promise followed by a disappointing follow-up is common to many of the 'exciting break-through' research headlines in the popular press. Some new research has now been done on the benefits of coconut oil in patients with Alzheimer's disease. After 21 days using a diet based on the well-known 'Mediterranean Diet' but enriched with coconut oil, improvements in cognitive function were seen.[9a] This small study noted definite improvement in orientation and sematic memory and recommended further studies be carried out. Unfortunately the first placebo-controlled trial of coconut oil was abandoned due to lack of sufficient participants but other trials have indicated a benefit from including coconut oil in the diet. Further trials are needed before any firm conclusions can be made.

Research has been done which involved using mice to test the effect of a high-fat, low-carbohydrate diet. The conclusion of this research stated: 'Here we demonstrate that a diet rich in saturated fats and low in carbohydrates can actually reduce levels of amyloid beta. Therefore, dietary strategies aimed at reducing amyloid beta levels should take into account inter-actions of dietary components and the metabolic outcomes, in particular, levels of carbohydrates, total calories, and presence of ketone bodies should be considered.'[10] Of course it needs to be remembered that not all animal-based research translates into benefits in humans.

A US-based, 90-day, randomised, double-blind, placebo-controlled, parallel-group study which involved giving people with early to moderate Alzheimer's (AD) an oral ketogenic compound resulted in significant differences in ADAS-Cog scores of those taking the compared with the placebo group. The authors concluded: 'Therefore, chronic induction of ketosis may offer a novel strategy for AD that can be used with current therapies.'[11] ('Ketosis' is the metabolic state we are in when we are using fats rather than glucose as our source of energy.)

Vitamins and nutritional supplements

The body also requires a supply of vitamins, minerals, trace elements and polyphenols to function correctly. The most common advice is that if the diet is adequate in respect of protein, fats and carbohydrates then a sufficient supply of these 'micro-nutrients' will be taken in. However, this is not necessarily true and much research has focused on the possible help that dietary supplements may provide in lowering the risk of dementia.

There have been a number of trials (see below) to test whether these supplements are effective in preventing dementia and whether they improve symptoms in those who already have dementia. A problem with such trials is the fact that any dietary supplementation takes time to show its effects. This means any trials have to be carried out over a long period of time. In addition, trials usually have to be carried out using specific supplements – perhaps in pill form – that make it easy for participants to take part. Trying to ensure that participants in a trial eat particular foods in sufficient quantities is much more difficult.

Given the fact that in general, vitamins and minerals are a part of a normal diet it can be quite difficult to design research that tests that any one supplement can make a difference to the risk of developing dementia. Indeed, two pieces of research maintain clearly that it is not possible to prove that supplements make any difference to those with normal cognition nor to identify any supplements which can reduce the risk of people with MCI developing dementia or which can effectively treat their symptoms.[12, 13]

Such evidence refers to normally healthy people without dietary deficiencies. Where there is a proven deficiency in the diet the case appears to be different.

B vitamins

Any general reference to B vitamins is complicated by the fact that since 'vitamin B' was first identified many diverse classes of this vitamin have been found, each of which is either a cofactor (a substance whose presence is essential) for key metabolic processes or is a precursor (a substance from which another is formed) needed to make one. Partly for this reason the various B vitamins are now often referred to by their names (for example, thiamine (B1) and folic acid (B9)).

Significant research has been carried out around folic acid. It has been noted that a rise in blood levels of a particular amino acid called homocysteine is associated with an increased risk of Alzheimer's disease and vascular dementia as well as stroke and heart disease. At the present time it is still not clear whether raised homocysteine levels are a pointer to an increased risk of dementia and heart disease (including stroke) or whether raised levels are *caused* by heart disease and dementia. Supplements of folic acid can be shown to lower levels of homocysteine in the blood and for a while this line of research appeared very exciting. However, clinical trials have shown that even when homocysteine levels are reduced this does not restore cognitive function in those people with early stage dementia, nor does it appear to improve the prognosis for those with cardiac problems. A systematic review (a type of secondary research which summarises large bodies of evidence) of vitamin supplementation and dementia was carried out in 2022 by Victoria Gil Martinez and colleagues and this looked at the effects of supplementation with folic acid, vitamin C, vitamin E and vitamin D. The findings of this systematic review suggest that supplementation of B-omplex vitamins, especially a supplementation of folic acid, may have a positive effect on delaying and preventing the risk of cognitive decline.[14]

Vitamin B12

Vitamin B12 plays a significant role in the human body, especially when it comes to nerve cells, brain cells and DNA functioning. It is naturally available mostly from animal products and a deficiency of B12 can be associated with symptoms such as confusion, depression, memory problems, fatigue and balance problems. Some of these symptoms can appear to be the same as those of dementia and so normally anyone presenting to the doctor with dementia symptoms will be given a blood test to show if there is a B12 deficiency which might be the cause of their symptoms.

Vitamin D

Some research has been carried out into the connection between low levels of vitamin D and dementia. Levels of this vitamin are often low in older people generally and are lower in the general population than a generation ago. The reason seems to be that the main source of vitamin D for the body is from the action of sunlight on the skin. Many older people, especially those living in residential care homes, may not go out into the sun very much. In addition, a great deal of publicity has been given to the connection between skin cancer and sunlight damage to skin and the use of sun-screen cream is much higher than it used to be. *The American Journal of Alzheimer's Disease and Other Dementias* reported in a paper published in 2011 that: 'Patients with Alzheimer's disease in particular have a high prevalence of vitamin D deficiency which is also associated with low mood and impaired cognitive performance in older people.' The authors noted that: 'Vitamin D clearly has a beneficial role in AD (Alzheimer's disease) and improves cognitive function in some patients with AD.'[15]

Given that current advice is to apply high-factor sunscreen and to avoid direct sunlight in the middle of the day (the time when the action of sun on the skin is most effective at producing vitamin D), this research finding is clearly very interesting, if perhaps, controversial.

Regarding vitamin D supplementation, the findings of the review discussed above noted that results vary vastly among different trials. This means that there is a lack of certainty in assessing the potential benefits that vitamin D might have on cognition.

Vitamin E

Vitamin E is an antioxidant, a substance that scientists believe may protect brain cells and other body tissues from certain kinds of chemical wear and tear. A 1997 study showed that high doses of vitamin E delayed loss of ability to carry out daily activities and placement in residential care for several months.[16]

The review of 2022 mentioned in the discussion on vitamin B12[14] also suggested that high dose-vitamin E supplementation had positive effects on cognition. However, scientists have found evidence in other studies that high-dose vitamin E may slightly increase the risk of death, especially for those with coronary artery disease.

Vitamin E in high doses can interact with some medications, including those prescribed to keep blood from clotting or to lower cholesterol. Therefore vitamin E supplements should be taken with caution and only after checking with your doctor.

Ginko biloba

Ginko biloba is a herbal supplement which has a reputation for improving learning and memory. Initial research published in 2002 seemed to show promise for application of its properties to help those diagnosed with dementia.[17] This was borne out by the reputation of the herb and its use by herbalists for the improvement of memory in students studying for examinations. However, in a later study published in the *Journal of the American Medical Association*, 240 milligrams per day of ginkgo biloba as a dietary supplement was found to be ineffective in reducing the development of dementia and Alzheimer's disease in older people. This study, known as the GEM (Ginko Evaluation of Memory) study, led by Steven T DeKosky, MD, is the largest clinical trial ever to evaluate ginkgo's effect on the occurrence of dementia.[18]

Some medical herbalists have claimed that the dose used in the trial was insufficient to achieve effective improvement and in fact a systematic review and meta-analysis of ginko-biloba in neuropsychiatric disorders *including* dementia (both Alzheimer's disease and vascular dementia) conducted in 2013 recommended the use of ginko-biloba in dementia and suggested that the effect was comparable to donepezil (the most commonly prescribed dementia drug).[19]

This meta-analysis did point out the variation in research results so unfortunately, clinical trials have not shown *consistently* (perhaps due to the dosage) that ginko helps to prevent cognitive loss in normal elderly subjects, or to improve cognitive function in patients already diagnosed with Alzheimer's disease, meaning that doctors are not convinced of any benefit from this supplement.

Essential minerals

Some minerals (such as calcium, iron and zinc) are essential for health. We need these minerals in varied amounts - some of them in very small amounts - but they are still essential and we can become ill if we do not get sufficient. Supplementing with minerals can be problematic because the interactions between minerals are complex. For example, too much calcium can interfere with zinc absorption. If you take large quantities of iron you will not be able to absorb zinc. If you are consuming a good and varied diet with the minimum of processed foods you should get all the amounts of minerals you need. Most multivitamin supplements also contain essential minerals.

Polyphenols

Polyphenols are bioactive phytochemicals found in plant foods, spices and beverages. They can act as antioxidants, meaning they can neutralise harmful free radicals that would otherwise damage your cells. They may help to improve health conditions including dementia. Some research has been done into the effect of polyphenols on preventing and treating dementia – especially on the benefits of drinking green tea – but this research suffers from the same problems of isolating substances in the diet, ensuring that certain items are consumed and reliance on self-reporting as all diet-related research. A paper published in the *Journal of Nutritional Biochemistry* concluded that though 'human polyphenol research on cognitive function is at an early stage and much work needs to be done, the observed associations are promising and call for future investigation.'[20]

Mushrooms

Mushrooms of all edible varieties are high in many of the B vitamins and if grown under ultra-violet light or outdoors will also be high in vitamin D. Many varieties also contain polyphenols that have antioxidant and anti-inflammatory properties that may be protective against neurodegeneration. Consequently, there has been a lot of new research around the role of mushrooms in the diet and the effect on cognition. Of particular interest for the subject of this book is the paper published in the *Journal of Alzheimer's Disease* in 2019. This research examined the association between mushroom intake and mild cognitive impairment (MCI) using data from 663 participants aged 60 and above, and concluded that people who consumed more than two portions of mushrooms per week were less likely to develop MCI irrespective of other risk factors such as education, cigarette smoking, heart disease or social activities.[21]

Diet after a diagnosis

If you have been diagnosed with dementia or if you are caring for someone with this diagnosis you can make useful changes to the diet that make it more nutrient-rich. You can switch to using full-fat milk and include plenty of eggs, cheese and butter. You can also include oily fish several times per week, though some people prefer a fish-oil supplement. You can ensure that you or the person you care for eats more unprocessed foods (for example, brown rice and wholemeal bread) and reduces their consumption of processed carbohydrates and hydrogenated fat.

Although research so far has not shown food supplements to be the magic answer to dementia there is no reason why you should not include supplements in the diet *provided you follow recommended guidelines*. So, for example, if you want to include a multi-vitamin or coconut oil or ginko biloba in the diet, this is unlikely to be harmful.

People in the later stages of dementia often lose weight so it is then even more important to ensure that whatever they eat is nutrient-rich. If weight loss is significant, food can be fortified and advice on the best way to manage this can be obtained, in the UK, from the Community Mental Health Team or a dementia support worker.

Conclusion

This chapter has looked at some of the discussion around diet and dementia prevention as well as considering current thinking about what constitutes a healthy diet. For specific advice about using diet to prevent dementia and dietary actions you can take now to decrease your risk, please refer to Chapter 9.

PART II

Assessing personal risk factors

In Part II of this book we will be looking at personal risk factors and assessing our personal 'current status' with regard to what is known at this time about the risk of dementia.

This part of the book is not supposed to be a kind of 'tick list' with a score of our individual risk profile but more a chance for you, the reader, to assess your own lifestyle and how this corresponds to what is currently known about increased risk of cognitive impairment.

It is important to bear in mind that current knowledge is still limited and, just as we have all heard of the heavy lifelong smoker who lived to be 100 with no lung disease, many of us know a grandparent who perhaps could tick all the boxes for raised risk factors and kept a razor-sharp mind until death.

However, if you are serious about trying to dodge dementia, then it makes sense to assess your current situation with regard to the various risk factors before reading in Part III the details of what steps you could take to reduce your risk insofar as our current knowledge suggests.

Chapter 6

Assessing personal risk factors

Genetics and your personal history of trauma, mental health problems and physical disease

- The ApoE4 gene is associated with an increased risk of developing Alzheimer's disease and its presence can be identified with a simple blood test.
- Although we cannot change our past, we can by various means come to terms with it and strengthen our ability to deal with the traumatic life events that will inevitably come our way.
- Specific chronic health problems are known to be associated with increased risk of developing dementia, including:
  - Type 2 diabetes
  - Underactive thyroid
  - Lupus erythematosus
  - Rheumatoid arthritis
  - Hearing loss if not corrected
  - Age-related macular degeneration.
- Medications prescribed 'preventatively' may have dementia-like side effects so weigh up their benefits and drawbacks.
- Certain vitamin deficiencies can be associated with dementia-like symptoms.

- Increased risk is not the same as certainty so reducing the risk is worth considering if you are serious about dodging dementia.

The previous chapters have discussed the evidence, as far as it is known, for various risk factors which might predispose us to develop dementia caused by Alzheimer's disease, vascular problems, Lewy bodies or other issues. Assessing individual risk is always going to be rather nebulous since there are many confounding factors with any disease. For example, there are many cases of people diagnosed with 'terminal' cancer who go on to live for many years more than predicted by their doctors. There are heavy smokers who never suffer from lung cancer. Dr Jerry Thomson's book *Curing The Incurable: Beyond The Limits of Medicine* gives many instances of people who, by all conventional medical knowledge, should have died from their ailments and have not.[1] However, my book is specifically about trying to avoid developing dementia and so we will look now at how to try to assess personal risk factors and (in Part III), how to mitigate these risks.

Genetics: ApoE4

Certain genes can affect a person's risk of developing Alzheimer's disease, in particular although our knowledge about this is incomplete. The evidence for a genetic cause is clearer for younger-onset than for late-onset Alzheimer's disease.

Early-onset Alzheimer's disease and genetics

The three genes that have a major effect on the risk of developing Alzheimer's disease are the amyloid precursor protein (APP) gene and two presenilin genes (PSEN-1 and PSEN-2). People with any of these genes tend to develop the disease in their 30s or 40s, and come from families in which several members also have/had early-onset Alzheimer's disease.

If you have early-onset familial Alzheimer's disease due to this genetic defect, you will already know about this at an early age and these chapters are not strictly relevant to you. You can get more information and support from Dementia UK at: (www.dementiauk.org/youngonset).

Later-onset Alzheimer's disease and genetics

With late-onset dementia, the pattern is not so clear. For example, a gene called apolipoprotein E (ApoE) has been shown to play a part in the development of late-onset Alzheimer's disease and vascular dementia. (It has been mentioned in several of the earlier chapters.) The effects of various combinations of the ApoE gene seem to be subtle and, although it is not believed that these directly cause Alzheimer's, the variations seem to increase or decrease the risk of developing the disease.

This gene comes in three forms, or 'alleles'. Because we inherit one ApoE gene from our mother and another from our father, we each have two copies of this gene and these may be the same as each other or different, meaning that each of us can inherit a number of possible combinations. The names and effects of the three variants are as follows:

- ApoE2: This form of the gene is mildly protective against the development of Alzheimer's disease. Altogether, 11% of the population is thought to have one copy of ApoE2 together with a copy of ApoE3, and one in 200 to have two copies of ApoE2.
- ApoE3: About 60% of the population has two copies of the ApoE3 gene and they have an 'average risk' which means about half of this group develop Alzheimer's

disease by their late 80s.

- ApoE4: The ApoE4 gene is associated with a higher risk of Alzheimer's. About a quarter of the population inherits one copy of this gene. This increases their risk of developing Alzheimer's disease by up to four times. About 2% of the population inherits two copies of the ApoE4 gene – one from each parent – which means they are at 10 times the risk of developing Alzheimer's disease.

As research on the genetics of Alzheimer's disease progresses, researchers are uncovering links between late-onset Alzheimer's and a number of other genes.

A blood test can identify which ApoE alleles a person has, but results cannot predict who will or will not develop Alzheimer's disease. Currently, ApoE testing is used primarily in research settings to identify study participants who may have an increased risk of developing Alzheimer's.

Knowing that you have an increased risk of developing dementia may be considered helpful by some people but others would rather not know. It is important to remember that 'increased risk' does not mean certainty.

Personal history of trauma and mental health issues

In Chapter 2 we discussed the increased risk associated with trauma, mental health issues and physical diseases experienced in the past. If you have experienced some of these issues and, after reading this chapter, have perhaps felt that things are stacked against you and that the risks are so high that it is inevitable that you will develop dementia, it is important to remember that risk factors are just that – they are factors that increase the risk. They are not certainties.

Another thing to bear in mind is that many people experience trauma, mental health issues and serious physical disease and they do not go on to develop dementia. As far as we can tell it seems that it is not the actual experience of these issues that increases the risk of developing dementia but the way in which these issues are dealt with, the way the body responds and ultimately the residual effects, that may cause a continuing stress on the mind or body.

Take trauma, for example. As pointed out in Chapter 2, few of us escape physical injury of some kind in our lives, and although not all of us have to manage severe mental health issues we all have to deal with emotional challenges, upsetting events and the death of someone close to us – perhaps a parent or friend or sibling.

Remember that research and experience are beginning to suggest that it is not the actual experience of trauma that possibly triggers dementia but the way in which each one of us manages to deal with the experience and the outcomes of traumatic events.

In my work I have been frequently struck by the number of newly diagnosed individuals who list a history of recent trauma – not just one event but often a series of traumatic events following swiftly one after another. It may be illness, death of a loved one, a calamitous event or a mixture of several of these. It is as if the human mind can deal with stressful and traumatic occurrences to a certain extent but that there comes a tipping point. Obviously this tipping point is different for each person and to a certain extent is governed by the amount and the kind of support received.

Research into the effects of trauma on mental health

The term 'shell shock', which was coined by Dr Charles Myers in

1916, was later called 'battle fatigue', but the experience is much more complex. After some initial bewilderment on the part of the medical authorities, it was concluded that constant stress from battle was the cause of the strange 'nervous symptoms' experienced by some soldiers. The symptoms are now known as post-traumatic stress disorder (PTSD).

Interestingly, doctors identified during the First World War that soldiers with a stable and supportive childhood background were less likely to succumb to 'shellshock'. It did not seem to be a question of the level of support received after the appearance of symptoms but rather the fact that those who had experienced a supportive and stable childhood and early adolescence seemed better able to deal with the constant level of stress resulting from their time in the trenches.

More recently, Bessel Van Der Kolk in his book *The Body Keeps the Score* emphasised how early life experiences can influence the ability to deal with later mental trauma. Those who experienced abuse or neglect in childhood and who found it difficult to feel 'safe' in any environment were the people most likely to suffer mental ill-health in later life and to turn to alcohol or drugs to cope with everyday life.[2]

Lucy Easthope, a leading authority on recovering from disaster, describes vividly how the way in which traumatic events are dealt with by authority figures can affect the ability of people to recover from a calamitous event.[3]

When we consider research such as the above it can seem as though the ability to come through trauma and tragedy and remain mentally stable is out of our hands – based in the history of our past. However, there are many other factors to consider. It is salutary to learn about the difficulties that many famous and not-so-famous people have overcome in their lives. Some of the factors that have been identified which enable people to come to terms with the past and to 'rise above' the outcomes are:

- Having a present loving and supportive relationship

- Being part of a caring and supportive community
- Having a strong spiritual belief
- Being able to understand the reason for and to forgive past wrongs
- Being able to channel negative feelings into positive actions
- Being given the right professional therapeutic help and support.

It is clear from the above list that, although we cannot change our past, we can by various means come to terms with it and strengthen our ability to deal with the traumatic life events that will inevitably come our way.

A personal history of past ill health and disease

It may be that the same factors apply to the effects of past physical disease.

We looked in Chapter 2 at the effects of physical disease on the risk of dementia in later life. Some childhood diseases were considered to be far more serious in the past than they are today and were treated accordingly. Measles and mumps, for example, involved bedrest and a three-week quarantine from others in the 1950s and 1960s and often a period of 'convalescence' afterwards. Partly this was because the medical treatment was less advanced and partly because there was less knowledge about the spread of disease. It may also be true that the nutritive status and thus the robustness of children was lower in the past.

Treatment of disease was often different in the earlier part of the 20th century and clients have often told me of traumatic hospital stays, long periods of isolation and bewilderment at being separated from companions and family, especially parents. We might consider on reflection that the treatment was more of a risk factor for later health problems than the actual disease and reflect on the potential impact of lockdowns in the recent pandemic on people of all ages.

Every period has its signature disease and the early part of the 20th century was blighted by fear of tuberculosis (TB). In the 19th century many people were infected with TB by drinking milk from infected cattle. During the first half of the 1900s the risk of transmission from this source was dramatically reduced after the application of the pasteurisation process. By the 1950s, mortality in Europe had decreased by about 90%. Improvements in sanitation, vaccination and other public-health measures began significantly reducing rates of TB even before the arrival of effective antibiotics, although the disease remained a significant threat.[4] In 1946 the development of the antibiotic streptomycin made effective treatment and cure of TB a reality. (Interestingly there is a theory that TB and dementia are not only linked but are one and the same disease.)[5]

The treatment for TB, before antibiotics had been discovered, consisted often of long periods in a sanatorium or in hospital and separation from family and loved ones. Once again the traumatic effects of the treatment might result in later health problems.

Personal experience: One client of mine when dementia was first diagnosed spent a long time ruminating on the long spells in hospital that he had spent as a child, separated from his family and, at the time, not understanding why. It was hard to get him to come to terms with his dementia because he started to associate it with the treatment of his childhood illness.

The scourge of the mid-20th century was poliomyelitis (polio). Some who experienced this disease escaped lightly with a mild fever and some muscular aches but others were left incapacitated for life. Poliomyelitis has become newsworthy again more recently with the recognition of 'post-polio syndrome' where those who suffered from polio in the past have experienced a milder form of fatigue and muscular aches postulated to be a recurrence of the original infection.

Some suggestion has been made that cognitive problems are associated with post-polio syndrome but research has not so far confirmed this.

Few of us reach mid-life without some compromise to our health, even if it is only something like imperfect sight, dental problems, a tricky digestion or back problems. Which of us can claim never to have had a day of sickness or a minor health problem? Many people will have experienced a major health problem such as a serious illness or injury.

We have already seen how previous serious illness or injury can affect us for life and discussed how the experience of this must be taken into account when assessing the risk of experiencing dementia in the future. We should now look at other factors – many of which seem to have no bearing on dementia but, as we have discussed, all health factors are significant in this respect.

Relevant chronic diseases

There are many people who have health problems such as an autoimmune disease or chronic health problems who are able to manage these on an everyday basis and who are able to live a normal life whilst managing their symptoms. Some diseases and health problems are known to pre-dispose to dementia; for others there is no direct evidence of an effect but they may contribute to a poorer health outcome overall.

A few diseases are known to result in dementia as they progress – for example, HIV/AIDS, Creutzfeldt–Jakob disease (CJD), supranuclear palsy, Korsakoff's syndrome and Binswanger's disease. Some people with multiple sclerosis, motor neurone disease, Parkinson's disease or Huntington's disease may develop dementia as a result of the progression of neurodegeneration.

Type 2 diabetes

Diabetes is a very significant health issue and both type 1 and type 2 diabetes are known to contribute to a high risk of developing dementia. Type 2 diabtetes is also an increasingly common health condition.

A growing body of research links both type 1 and type 2 diabetes with both Alzheimer's disease and vascular dementia. There is even a school of thought which suggests that Alzheimer's disease is actually a third type of diabetes (see Chapter 2).

Type 2 diabetes has specifically been identified as a significant risk factor for age-related cognitive impairment, cognitive decline and dementia.[7] It has been demonstrated that people with mild cognitive impairment (MCI) who also have diabetes are three times more likely to develop dementia than those who have MCI alone.[8] There is evidence that patients who have type 2 diabetes are more likely to suffer cognitive impairment following a stroke than those patients who do not have diabetes.

The connection between dementia and type 2 diabtetes has been more fully discussed in Chapter 2.

Comorbidities

'Comorbities' is a term which many of us became familiar with during the Covid-19 pandemic. It simply means the presence of more than one disease or medical condition in an individual. So, we might use that term in connection with someone who has dementia and (for example) diabetes. When assessing your risk of developing dementia, any existing disease or chronic medical condition needs to be taken into account and this is why I have used the umbrella term comorbidity. It may be that you have only one pre-existing medical condition and so this is strictly speaking not a 'comorbidity', but in terms of discussing the risk factors it is convenient to use this term.

Some medical conditions are known to raise the risk factor of dementia – diabetes is one example, as discussed. However, there is every possibility that any factor which stresses the body either physically or mentally will make us more susceptible to dementia. Since we cannot pinpoint actual causes yet, any existing medical condition may be a risk factor.

Thyroid problems

According to a study reported in *Science Daily* and published in full in the 6 July 2022, online issue of *Neurology*, the medical journal of the American Academy of Neurology, older people with hypothyroidism (sometimes known as underactive thyroid), may be at increased risk of developing dementia.[9] The risk of developing dementia was even higher for people whose thyroid condition required thyroid hormone replacement medication.

Hypothyroidism occurs when the thyroid gland doesn't make enough thyroid hormones. This can slow metabolism. Symptoms include feeling tired all the time despite normal levels of sleep, weight gain, hair loss and over-sensitivity to cold. The study suggests that: 'people should be aware of thyroid problems as a possible risk factor for dementia and therapies that could prevent or slow irreversible cognitive decline.'

In this study, researchers looked at the health records of 7843 people newly diagnosed with dementia in Taiwan and compared them with the same number of people who did not have dementia. Their average age was 75. Researchers looked to see who had a history of either hypothyroidism or hyperthyroidism. Hyperthyroidism is when the thyroid produces too much hormone. This can increase metabolic rate.

Symptoms include unintended weight loss, rapid or irregular heartbeat and nervousness or anxiety.

Of the people with dementia, 68 or 0.9%, had hypothyroidism, compared with 34 of the people without dementia, or 0.4%. When researchers adjusted for other factors that could affect the risk of dementia, such as sex, age, high blood pressure and diabetes, they found that people over age 65 with hypothyroidism were 80% more likely to develop dementia than people of the same age who did not have thyroid problems.

The researchers found no link between hyperthyroidism and dementia and they also found that, for those aged under 65, having a history of hypothyroidism was not associated with an increased risk of dementia.[9]

In another paper, published in the Egyptian Journal of Internal Medicine,[10] researchers found 'a close correlation between thyroid status and cognitive dysfunction'. They suggested that thyroid function was associated with cognitive impairments induced by subcortical ischaemic vascular dementia (SIVD) and concluded that: 'thyroid dysfunction, especially subclinical hypothyroidism, is associated with cognitive impairment. Dementia increases more with more increase in TSH, and the MMSE score decreases with the increase of age.'[10] (TSH, or thyroid stimulating hormone, levels are used as an index of thyroid function as the body pumps out more TSH to try to stimulate greater thyroxin production when this is too low.)

Lupus

Systemic lupus erythematosus (SLE) is a chronic autoimmune disease affecting a wide range of body systems including the peripheral and central nervous system. The symptoms vary from person to person and may be mild or, in some cases, severe. Common symptoms include painful and swollen joints, fever, chest pain, hair loss, mouth ulcers, swollen lymph nodes, feeling tired and a red rash which is most commonly on the face (often called a 'butterfly rash' because of the shape).

Research published in the journal *Geriatric Psychiatry* in 2017 pointed to an association between lupus and dementia.[11] This study concluded that the proportion of people with dementia was higher amongst those who had SLE compared with controls without SLE. The study concluded that: 'Systemic lupus erythematosus is significantly associated with dementia. This finding should give rise to search for SLE in patients with an ambiguous cause for dementia, especially those with an early onset cognitive decline.'[11]

Another study, this time from Korea, determined that a diagnosis of SLE resulted in being 2.4 times more likely to develop dementia even after excluding other comorbidities.[12] The study used a database of individuals who had submitted medical claims from 2002 to 2013. It concluded that SLE significantly increased dementia risk regardless of type.

However, results from this same study suggest the risk for SLE patients is 15 times higher for early vascular dementia. The authors stated that: 'We believe that providing treatment to control disease activity, along with risk factor management, may help prevent dementia in SLE patients.'[12]

Rheumatoid arthritis

A study published in 2020 in the journal *Cureus* explored the relationship between rheumatoid arthritis (RA) and dementia.[13] It reviewed peer-reviewed articles on rheumatoid arthritis and dementia sourced from reputable databases such as Research Gate, National Center for Biotechnology Information, PubMed and Google Scholar. It mentioned that both diseases are associated with older persons and genetic factors and pointed out that the inflammation associated with rheumatoid arthritis reduces blood flow to vital body organs, which increases the risk of developing dementia. Additionally, the study revealed that medications used by RA patients increased the risk of developing dementia. Importantly, however, it was pointed out that biological therapies such as tumour necrosis factor (TNF) inhibitors can lower the risk of dementia.[13]

Hearing loss

Research over many years has shown a strong link between hearing loss and dementia. There is no evidence that hearing loss in itself *causes* dementia, but older people with hearing loss are significantly more likely to experience dementia than those whose hearing is not impaired. For some time, the main reasons for this link were considered to be the social isolation that can result from untreated hearing loss. However, a new theory suggests that the link may have something to do with the way the brain works. When someone is hard of hearing, they are often straining to hear and the effort involved can over-exert the brain, so that more mental energy is being used just to hear normal conversation. This particularly affects the temporal lobes of the brain.

The temporal lobes are the area of the brain where hearing is processed. They are also involved in vision, sensory input, language, emotion, comprehension — and in housing memories. If energy is diverted to hearing, then less energy is available to devote to memory, understanding and other cognitive functions.

One conclusion from this suggestion is that any aids to hearing will be helpful in decreasing the dementia risk. Firstly, you should protect your hearing – wear ear defenders if using noisy machinery and keep the volume turned down when listening to music. Try to have conversations with others in a quiet environment so that you are not straining to hear. If attending talks or lectures, do not allow pride to prevent you from choosing a front seat if your hearing is less than perfect.

Personal experience: I have experienced this as a presenter – I always request that anyone hard of hearing sits in the front seats, but many refuse to do so claiming that their hearing is not impaired and they then complain that they cannot hear me!

Secondly, if your hearing is impaired – and most older people have some hearing loss – then use the aids that are available. There are many types of hearing aid now so that even those who have sensitive ears (and are unable to bear anything in the ear) can benefit. People who successfully wear hearing aids have told me that it can take several weeks to get used to a new device but that eventually you do become unaware of them. The same people also tell me that hearing aids really can make a difference to your social enjoyment of life.

Age-related macular degeneration (AMD)

Scientists have known for some time that there is a connection between AMD and Alzheimer's disease.

Researchers noticed that AMD and Alzheimer's disease had factors in common. While both diseases are related to age, they also both are related to protein deposits and breakdown of neurones (nerve cells). People with AMD are more likely to have cognitive impairment, or trouble with thinking and communicating well, than patients without AMD.

While physicians are not sure why these diseases are linked, they do recognise that there is some relationship between AMD and Alzheimer's disease.

In a 2019 study aimed at determining the association between dementia and age-related macular degeneration (AMD) using meta-analysis, researchers found that AMD was associated with increased risk of AD/cognitive impairment and that patients with AMD had poorer cognitive functions when compared with controls. They noted 'a significant association between dementia/AD and AMD'.[14]

Physical disease in general

We see from the above that many physical diseases can be seen to increase the risk factor for developing dementia. It is difficult to establish the degree to which having one of these health conditions might increase the risk of being diagnosed with dementia in later life for any one individual. However, any pre-existing condition contributes to, and is indicative of, a poorer health status which increases the stress on the body and ultimately the brain.

Prescribed medications

We should now consider the effect of medication on the risk of dementia. It is estimated that the average person aged over 60 years is routinely taking at least four different medications. Most people taking such medications would consider themselves as healthy, so why are they taking the drugs? The simple answer is generally because they have been prescribed by the doctor. In other words, the drugs are what is generally described as 'preventative medicine' – medicine taken to prevent the possible development of an ill-health condition or a disease. This is essentially a modern phenomenon. It seems that most of us consider that the 'doctor knows best' and do not question whether a preventative drug might have a harmful effect upon our health. However, as Dr Jerry Thomson points out in Chapter 4 on Drugs and dementia, there can be side effects to some commonly prescribed drugs and some of those side effects can affect cognition – they can give us dementia-like symptoms.

> **Personal experience:** I was running a support group for carers – there were about 10 people present. When I mentioned the two drugs Jerry Thomson expresses concerns about in Chapter 4 – statins and proton pump inhibitors (PPIs) – almost all those attending said that they were taking one or both drugs. More importantly, not one of them said that they would ask the doctor whether the prescription was still necessary or ask about side effects. The interesting thing is that these were carers of people with dementia who were experiencing first-hand the problems encountered after a diagnosis.

If you have a medical condition that requires regular medication, then of course you should take this medication and follow your doctor's advice. You should, however, be made aware of any possible side effects and of any interactions with other medications. If your doctor does not mention these, you should ask him/her and also read the information that comes with all medications. Do not conclude that the doctor will automatically tell you about this. For one thing, doctors are busy and they are human. They might forget to mention something to you during the consultation. Or they might believe that any side effects are likely to be negligible and that you would be sure to ask about them should they occur.

If you are prescribed a long-term medication, then this prescription is supposed to be reviewed at regular intervals by your doctor. In addition, you can yourself ask the pharmacist to look at your medication and advise whether it needs reviewing. This is an area in which you should be proactive and take responsibility for your own health.

Suppose you are taking a medication that is vital for your

wellbeing but there are side effects that may cause dementia (or dementia-like symptoms)? This does not mean that you have to just cross your fingers and hope for the best. You can discuss with your GP or specialist doctor whether there is an alternative drug available or perhaps whether the dose can be changed. You can at least ask to be regularly monitored for any cognitive problems.

The situation is different for drugs which are given under the guise of 'health prevention'. For example, we might consider drugs such as statins which are given to lower cholesterol in otherwise healthy people because it is believed that a high cholesterol reading predisposes one to heart disease. In the case of drugs like these which are prescribed quite legally and with good intentions, it is up to the individual to assess the risk of accepting the prescription or not. There is no reason why you, as a concerned individual (concerned about your future health and the possibility of developing dementia), may not do your own research, ask questions of your GP or specialist and assess whether you prefer to take the risk of developing the medical problem which the drugs are supposed to prevent or the risk of developing dementia in later life.

Once again, it is important not to conclude that 'the doctor knows best' because what we are talking about here is NOT medication that is essential for a life-threatening medical condition. We are talking about a medication that is being prescribed because it *might* help to protect you against developing illness in the years to come.

Interestingly, very few people prescribed a 'preventative medicine' bother to ask the doctor what the benefits might be, what the side effects might be and whether taking the medication actually improves the odds of dying at an earlier age than might otherwise be the case. As Dr Jerry Thomson has pointed out (see page 59), some of these prescribed drugs may actually *increase* the chance of developing dementia symptoms. You might like to consider discussing with your doctor the benefits of taking the drug weighed against the cost of developing dementia. Please do not forget that the final decision whether to take any medication rests with you and not with your doctor.

Vitamin deficiencies

Another area of present health which is worth consideration is that of vitamin deficiency. The Covid-19 crisis raised awareness of this when it became clear that those with ultra-low vitamin D status were more likely to contract Covid-19 and also more likely to have a poor outcome if they did become infected. Vitamin status is an area which should definitely be addressed if you are considering looking at avoiding dementia in later life and we go into this in more depth in the chapter on Nutrition. However, the B vitamins (and particularly vitamin B12 status) deserve special consideration. Low levels of B12 can result in depression and mental confusion similar to some symptoms of dementia. In theory, if you present to your GP with suspected dementia, your vitamin B levels should be one of the standard 'elimination' blood tests that will be done routinely, but many of my clients have told me that this had not been done. In any case, the standard blood test for vitamin B12 deficiency may not indicate if there is a deficiency because individual requirements can vary.

Be aware also that certain commonly-prescribed drugs can lead to B12 deficiency. These include proton pump inhibitors such as omeprazole, and metformin prescribed for type 2 diabetes and 'pre-diabetes'. Gastric atrophy with age, and GI surgery can also cause B12 deficiency without patients being warned: (https://pernicious-anaemia-society.org/b12deficiency andperniciousanaemia/).

Remember that it is possible to have blood tests done privately in the UK and the cost is not exorbitant so if your GP will not cooperate you can take matters into your own hands in this respect at least.

Conclusion

At the end of this chapter we come back to the important point that risk, even very high risk, and certainty are two different things. However, if you are serious about dodging dementia, it is important to consider how many of the above risks factors apply to you, or the person you are concerned about, and therefore the relative importance of mitigating risk wherever this is within your control.

Chapter 7

Assessing your current status

Important risk factors to consider include:
- Lifestyle, nutrition, exercise, social inclusion, work/ leisure balance
- . MCI (mild cognitive impairment)
- Particular concerns
- Family history
- Caring for someone with dementia.

As described in the Introduction, a report in *The Lancet* published in 2020 stated that modifying 12 risk factors might prevent or delay up to 40% of dementias.[1]

We have discussed assessing personal risk with regard to past and ongoing physical and mental illness, past trauma and medication. In this chapter we consider your current status in respect of lifestyle habits and behaviours, nutrition, exercise regimes and social inclusion. We will then consider particular concerns – for example, whether you already have mild cognitive impairment (MCI), whether you have concerns about your memory and cognition and what your family history is with regard to dementia.

Lifestyle

The umbrella term 'lifestyle' could cover all the items in the rest of this chapter but here I am using it to consider some lifestyle habits and behaviours which were discussed in full in Chapter 3 as well as nutrition discussed in Chapter 5. Most of us have some features of our lifestyle which are not considered to be 'good' or healthy. Perhaps we smoke, drink too much alcohol, forget to exercise and eat too much of the 'wrong' foods. Often it seems that all the things which we enjoy, which make life 'worth living' are forbidden and bad for us.

The point of this chapter is to assess our current status with regards to dementia risk. At this stage do not lose heart if you feel that you have lifestyle habits which raise your risk and which you feel unable or unwilling to address. The simple facts are that – as far as current research can show:

- Smoking is bad for your general health and it raises the risk of dementia.
- Evidence about alcohol intake is more equivocal but current research indicates that drinking no alcohol and drinking more than the recommended guidelines both raise your risk of dementia.
- Being obese raises your risk of developing dementia.
- Using illegal recreational drugs is a general health risk and some (such as cannabis) raise your risk of dementia.
- Polypharmacy (taking a large number of prescribed drugs) raises your risk of dementia.

Smoking, alcohol intake and the part played by prescribed drugs have been discussed in earlier chapters in some detail. We discuss some specific risk factors in more detail below.

Your diet and nutritional status

Let us look first at nutritional status. The details are addressed in Chapters 5 and 10 but this section is to prompt you to think about what your current diet actually is.

The facts about nutrition and its role in preventing dementia were extensively discussed in Chapter 5 together with some of the evidence base for this and some of the research studies that have been conducted. The problem is that current media coverage is biased away from this research, and it is easy to be beguiled by the latest book, the weekly news article, the current 'fad' diet. In Chapter 10 we will consider some of these ideas and look at the evidence behind them.

The diet most highly recommended by the medical press is the Mediterranean diet. Our grandparents would probably recognise this diet as the 'good mixed diet' which was promulgated in their youth.

The one area where there is general agreement amongst clinicians is obesity. If you are obese it is bad for your physical and mental health. One of the recommendations in the *Lancet Report* quoted at the beginning of this chapter concerns obesity.[1] There is evidence to support the relationship between increased body mass index (BMI) and dementia. A review of 19 longitudinal studies (that's studies that follow individuals over a long time) included 589,649 people aged 35 to 65 years, followed up for up to 42 years. It reported obesity (but not merely being overweight) was associated with late-life dementia.[2] If you are obese – or even overweight – then general medical opinion as well as research suggests that you should address this.

If you feel at present that you have a rather good diet, consider how you arrived at that conclusion. Is your diet similar to that of your friends and family? Are you influenced in what you eat by the latest news articles? (Of course you are!) Are you still eating the 'heart friendly' diet which you began to eat in mid-life – even after reading Chapter 5 of this book? Are you diabetic and if so have you changed your diet and eating habits to accommodate this? Do you suffer from indigestion more than occasionally? If so, do you take medication prescribed by your doctor? (See Jerry Thomson's advice in Chapter 4.) Have you cut foods out of your diet because they 'no longer agree with you'? If you do not feel that your diet keeps you in the best of health, how much are you willing to change your eating habits and how easy will this be if you are living with a partner of other family members?

In considering your current nutritional status then, think about how much you are influenced by the media and how likely it is that you will feel able to change your eating habits *even in order to avoid dementia*. This is the hardest factor to tackle. Dementia can seem far away and the constant barrage from the newspapers, TV, magazines, websites and podcasts can be insidious.

Physical exercise

Let us consider next the vexed question of physical exercise. Interestingly, research studies show conflicting results about the benefit of exercise on people who actually have dementia,[1] but physical exercise is known to be good for cardiovascular health.

Some people are enthusiastic about exercise and some shudder at the very word. But exercise does not have to mean wearing lycra and sweating it out in a gym. You may be surprised to be told that gardening, walking, bowls, golf, housework, carrying shopping and some forms of DIY are all forms of exercise.

Any form of exercise is better than none at all. The real emphasis is on movement. Some people favour gentle movement such as pilates and tai chi and some prefer running or active sport. It is generally considered that it is important to do some form of exercise which makes you breathless at least once a week, but this might be something as simple as walking or dancing.

The fact is that as we get older we tend to exercise less. This may be to do with disabling aches and pains such as those caused by arthritis or it may simply be inertia. It can come about because the people we used to exercise with (spouse, friend, neighbour) are no longer able to join us for one reason or another.

> **Covid note:** During the Covid crisis many people ceased to exercise because of gym closures, restrictions on and fear of going out and difficulty meeting other people and the closure of many local amenities such as parks. There was also a misunderstanding in the UK about government guidelines concerning exercise. I lost count of the clients who told me that one was only allowed to exercise for one hour a day which was nowhere specified in government guidelines.

Check current health guidelines on exercise and decide whether you currently are physically active enough. If you are a bit of a 'couch potato' then are you worried *enough* about the prospect of developing dementia to change your habits? How fit are you now? You should not suddenly start a vigorous exercise regime if you are not reasonably fit already. Most exercise advice suggests you check with your doctor before you begin a new regime (although I suspect most GPs would be surprised if you booked an appointment for this purpose) and there are many exercise programmes which allow you to 'work your way up' from whatever level of fitness you have now. What are current guidelines on enough exercise?

Current exercise guidelines

NHS UK suggests that adults should do at least 150 minutes of moderate-intensity activity a week or 75 minutes of vigorous-intensity activity a week. This exercise should be spread evenly over four or five days a week. It is also suggested that to be healthy we should all reduce time spent sitting or lying down.

Now, 150 minutes sounds a lot until you break that down over the recommended five days per week; then it becomes about 30 minutes a day. Remember that walking, gardening and housework all count as exercise.

Some forms of physical exercise claim to actually address illness. Qigong, for example, is a Chinese system of holistic health practice which incorporates specific exercise patterns to maintain health and it is also used by many to cure specific conditions.

Consider then, your current state of physical fitness, whether you are prepared to improve your physical fitness and exercise more in order to try to prevent the development of dementia, and if so, what activities would be attractive enough to encourage you to keep to your resolution.

Social inclusion

Having social networks and interactions with others is a key factor in avoiding dementia. In this respect, the Covid-19 'lockdowns' and discouragement of social meetings had a specific and direct bad effect on those who either already had a diagnosis of dementia or were suffering from MCI. Only time will tell how many new cases of dementia can be laid at the door of the Covid-19 restrictions.

'Infrequent social contact' is one of the risk factors stated in the *Lancet Report* and it can be worthwhile to assess your 'social interaction' status if you are seriously thinking about avoiding dementia.

It is worth first thinking about all the people you know – your social networks – and considering how big a part these play in your current life.

Many friendships and acquaintances are made through our

work activities (that is our paid jobs) or through our children, and often these social contacts continue for many years, surviving changes of job, children growing up and differing circumstances. Other relationships fall away when we change job, move house or our children grow up and leave home.

Some social contacts are made through hobbies (walking groups, sports clubs) and shared interests or volunteering (church communities, Scouts and Guides, Rotary clubs) and these contacts may be reduced when we cease to take part in the shared activities. Conversely, some people find that the friendships they made through these activities outlive the activities themselves so that, for example, the friend you met when escorting your child to football matches is still a close companion although your football-mad child is now a grown person with children of their own.

Neighbours too, can play a part in our social interactions as can casual contacts such as the person who you get to know at the supermarket checkout, the delivery person who brings your mail, the dog walker you pass the time of day with, the allotment holder who rents the plot next door to yours and other people you may 'know' although you would not call them regular friends.

There seems to be a connection between being married (or in a long term partnership) and a lower risk of dementia. This is postulated to be because married people have a wider social circle and more social contacts rather than any benefit from the married state as such. A systematic review and meta-analysis of relevant research, including in total 812,047 people worldwide, found an elevated dementia risk in lifelong single and widowed people compared with married people and the association was consistent in different sociocultural settings.[3]

Loneliness is considered to be a huge problem in the older population and some specific associations have been set up to try to combat this (for example, The Silver Line who claim to 'offer friendship, conversation, and support to those who need it'), but there are many older people who have few friends and acquaintances and yet would not consider themselves to be lonely. People also vary in their interpretation of loneliness, which does not necessarily correspond to having few social contacts. Interestingly, loneliness is not associated with an increased risk of dementia but lack of social interaction is.[4]

Although research indicates that wide social networks and frequent social contact are associated with a reduced risk of developing dementia, it is almost impossible to itemise what the terms mean. Do we get more protection from meeting a lot of people at large social events or from frequently meeting fewer people? If loneliness is not a significant factor, is it sufficient to just chat to a wide range of people in a casual manner or should we be making efforts to deepen our friendships and have more intense relationships? Is it more important to have social contact with someone every day or to have 'meaningful' prolonged contact even if at less frequent intervals? Research does indicate that belonging to a social group, such as a club, church, or set of people who meet regularly, is an important protective factor but it is rather difficult to break down what elements of that 'belonging' are significant.

During the Covid-19 outbreak, a great deal of emphasis was placed on 'remote' social contact such as that using social media (Facebook, Twitter, etc) and technological 'meetings' (such as Zoom), and many found this both useful and effective to ensure the maintenance of contact with others. However, as soon as face-to-face meetings were permitted once more, it was clear that in general, people were relieved to resume that form of contact. It was also significant that (apart from some who were exceptionally afraid or felt they had to 'shield' due to severe ill-health), many people accepted a degree of discomfort and endured complicated arrangements in order to meet others. For example, many more people than usual met in groups outside even during cold and wet weather, and large numbers were prepared to take inconvenient and slightly unpleasant Covid tests in order to attend meetings, to travel or to meet up with others.

Covid note: One very interesting fact I came to realise which emerged in the welter of 'remote' meetings and conversations is that most people with any form of dementia are unable to use technology to maintain relationships. This is not simply because of the difficulty in manipulating technology and learning new systems but because of the difficulty for someone with dementia of understanding that the remote image and voice are in any way 'real'. Probably this should not have come as a surprise because even before Covid it was understood that, as dementia progressed, many of those with cognitive problems had difficulty coping with such things as telephone conversations, reflections in mirrors, television images and social media of many kinds.

The main conclusion to take from these experiences is perhaps that it is not social 'contact' (via telephone, email or remote meetings) that has most significance when trying to avoid dementia, but in-person social interaction – the physical seeing, speaking and interacting with others. If this is so, then the casual chat at the supermarket checkout, an exchange with a fellow dog-walker or with the delivery person, may be more useful for avoidance of dementia than a telephone call or social media post.

Work and leisure balance

Many people when the time comes to retire from full time employment make comprehensive plans to fill their 'spare' time with outings, trips away, volunteering and further learning opportunities. It is more rare to find someone contemplating spending their retirement 'doing nothing'. This would seem to indicate that people generally recognise the benefit to their physical and mental health of keeping themselves occupied and of having an aim and interest in their lives. Research has shown that having a sense of purpose lowers the risk of developing dementia. Results from a meta-analysis of relevant research revealed that purpose in life was significantly associated with a reduced risk of dementia,[5] but many people lose their purpose in life when they stop doing their job.

Just what do we define as a 'purpose in life'? For some this is centred around the family, caring for grandchildren, spending more time with family members and seeing that the future generation has 'a good start in life'. But we don't all have children and grandchildren and even those who have may not feel that their purpose in life centres around their family. Lifelong learning is attractive to many and such organisations as the University of the Third Age (u3a) plus the great opportunities now available to learn almost any subject using the internet make this a very valid and easy-to-access option. Many people find a purpose in life through volunteering or giving time and energy to a 'cause', but a purpose in life doesn't have to be grand – there are many retired people who give time and energy and achieve great satisfaction from something as simple as managing an allotment or garden and providing fresh vegetables and flowers to family and friends.

What seems to be important is that the 'life purpose' must be important to them, absorbing enough to need thought and planning and maintain a sense of being useful and perhaps also to be of benefit to others. Indeed, it is very significant that most of my clients who have dementia complain that they no longer feel useful and nothing seems to give them as much pleasure as being able to help others.

Particular concerns

Mild cognitive impairment (MCI)

In the past, MCI was not considered to be a 'diagnosis' but merely the name of a warning state, a bit like the 'pre-diabetic' term which is often used today to suggest that, whilst not actually diabetic, the person in question should be aware of the possibility of a diagnosis if lifestyle is not addressed. MCI was supposed to indicate that the person to whom it was applied had noticed and was worried about some symptoms which, whilst not actually severe enough to be classified as dementia, were abnormal and worrying.

These days I often have people coming to me for advice telling me that they have been 'diagnosed' with MCI and asking me how they can best help themselves to avoid dementia.

As stated in the Introduction, the term 'mild cognitive impairment' is used in connection with people who have worries about their cognition (or sometimes those whose relatives have worries about their cognition) but who, when tested using the standard tests for dementia, have not received a dementia diagnosis. There is no fixed level of cognition which draws a line in the sand stating that this person has dementia and this other person merely has MCI. In many ways it comes down to the opinion of the doctor carrying out the tests. However, the general agreement is that a person has MCI if they are finding more problems than previously encountered in managing their affairs but do *not* find that they unable to manage the activities of everyday living – shopping, domestic tasks, personal care, managing money, making and keeping appointments etc.

If you are reading this book because you have been told that you have MCI, then you may be looking at how you can ensure that your MCI does not degenerate into actual dementia and the next few chapters are critical for you.

Family history

You may be reading this book because you have discovered that there is a history of dementia in your family. In the past this might have been difficult to know about for several reasons. In the days when people tended to die at a relatively younger age than now, the early stages of dementia might have been missed, put down to 'old age' or kept hidden as something to be ashamed of. But times have changed, and not only is dementia more openly talked about, but people are beginning to notice the history of ill-health within the family and to investigate it.

The genetic connections of dementia used to be brushed aside because it was considered that only a very few and rare cases were connected with the inheritance of a faulty gene. Those who inherited this gene were thought to develop dementia at a young age and mostly to live in fairly 'closed' communities where having dementia in the later years was more common than not. Familial dementia is still a recognised (and rare) condition but research has now pinpointed that the genetic connection is also present in late-onset dementia, as was discussed in Chapter 6.

If you have a family history of dementia, you may be reading this book as a self-help guide; in that case, addressing any factors such as lifestyle, dealing with adverse life events, coming to terms with the effects of past illness and mitigating the effects of any long-term health conditions are all sensible and effective precautions.

Caring for someone with dementia

In Chapter 6 we discussed some research that indicated that those who are living with a partner/spouse who has dementia are at a higher risk of developing dementia themselves. Very often it is when we find ourselves having to care for someone with dementia that we begin to think about the possibility of it affecting ourselves and to consider if there are any steps we can take to prevent developing cognitive difficulties in later life.

Unless you work with those who have dementia and with those who care for them, as I do, it is very difficult to understand how all-encompassing this care needs to be. My clients have variously described it as follows:

- It is like having a toddler who you can never leave alone for one minute.
- I live in a constant state of stress.
- I try to plan ahead but I don't know what crisis the next week will bring.
- At the beginning I had no idea of how this would take over my thoughts.
- It has taken over my life.
- I just didn't realise how the companionship in our relationship would disappear.
- I don't feel like a wife any more but like a minder.
- As her personality disintegrates I feel my mother is slipping away from me.
- It is like being bereaved before you actually are.

Most people in this situation give some thought to what might happen if they get dementia themselves and to consider how they might be able to prevent this.

Conclusion

The aim of this chapter has been to encourage you to continue your assessment of your current status with regard to avoiding dementia. In Chapter 6 we looked at physical and mental illness and the effects of adverse life events from the past, all of which have a bearing on your risk of developing dementia in the future. Some of the things in our past, such as adverse life events and physical and mental trauma, cannot be changed, but our attitude to them can be and this may make a difference to how these factors affect our risk of developing dementia in the future. The purpose of this chapter is to focus on assessing your present status with regard to several risk factors which can be addressed and the modifying of which has been shown to make a significant difference to the risk of being diagnosed with any form of dementia. As I have said, with each factor, you will want consider how important it is to you to 'dodge dementia' and make relevant changes.

In the next chapters we will be looking at the evidence which suggests what factors you might feel need modifying, how much weight to give to the different factors and how to take action to improve your chances of dodging dementia in later life.

The key things to do are:

- Give up smoking if you possibly can (see Chapter 3)
- Reduce your alcohol intake if it exceeds current guidelines for older age.
- Consider your diet (see Chapters 5 and 10).
- Assess your exercise level (see recommendations on page 117).
- Think about your social life (especially whether it has been reduced due to Covid-19 and not since revived) and consider how you might increase your social interactions.
- If you have MCI, follow the advice in this book in Chapters 7, 9, and 11.
- If you suspect you have MCI, talk to your doctor.
- If you are caring for someone with dementia, consider your own health and accept any support available.

PART III

What *you* can do now to dodge dementia

Having looked at some of the evidence for the various risk factors for developing dementia – insofar as we know them at present – in Part I and then discussed how we can evaluate our individual health and social situation in Part II, in this, the third section of the book we are going to concentrate on actions that you can take now to reduce your riskof developing dementia in the future.

Not everyone will feel compelled to take all these actions – or indeed any of them. Perhaps you will feel that since knowledge about the causes of dementia is still patchy at best you are happy to leave things to chance. Part III merely makes some suggestions for actions you can take now or in the near future. The rest is up to you.

Note that this section does not make suggestions concerning medication as this subject is covered in Chapter 4 (Dr Jerry Thompson's contribution).

Chapter 8

Nutrition: What should I eat?

Key points:
- There are many different diets with claims to change health but clear evidence for the claims is elusive.
- Extreme (omitting particular food groups) diets are not recommended.
- Some simple positive changes can be made to what we eat without too much difficulty.

A lot has been written about the role of nutrition in caring for those who have dementia but rather less about the role of nutrition in dementia prevention. This is not surprising because, although the general public is interested in nutrition, diet and the role of different food in connection with disease and wellbeing, the medical profession as a whole seem to be less so. Many doctors seem to regard attempts to treat illness through diet as akin to witch-doctoring and dismiss patient enquiries about the subject. When it comes to the prevention of ill health we find that many doctors are still giving out advice about low fat 'heart healthy' diets based on research which has now been shown to be out-of-date and possibly erroneous.

Is there a diet which helps to prevent dementia? As you might imagine, opinions on this are very varied and it can be highly confusing to try to find your way through the myriad of advice. Let us look at some of the 'health promoting' diets currently popular in the media.

Low-fat diet

The low-fat diet has been promoted for many years on the basis that saturated fat (of the kind found in meat and animal products) is bad for you because it increases your LDL ('bad') cholesterol, which in turn increases your risk of developing heart disease. This theory began with a hypothesis by Ancel Keys, a biologist and pathologist who, back in the 1930s, became persuaded that cholesterol was the main culprit in the development of heart disease and that the consumption of fat caused cholesterol to rise in the bloodstream. This idea was taken up by scientific and medical opinion and became firmly embedded in nutritional guidelines throughout the Western world. Indeed, despite later research (the Helsinki Businessmen Study, the Framingham study, the MRFIT trial and others) showing the errors in the fat-heart-health hypothesis, many people even today believe that the low-fat diet is THE healthy diet. As stated above, many doctors and nutritional websites still promote this diet.

As noted in Chapter 5, we need a steady intake of fat for the brain to function properly. Fats make up 60% of the brain and the nerves that run every system in the body. A low-fat diet is unlikely to reduce your risk of developing dementia. If you are overweight, it may help to cut down on fats in the diet but only in proportion to other food factors. In other words, those who are overweight should cut down on *everything*. Eating less fat will not help you to lose weight if in order to 'fill up' you eat more carbohydrate. The low-fat diet is an associate or off-shoot of the 'low-cholesterol diet'.

Low-cholesterol diet

As with the low-fat diet, the idea behind diets low in cholesterol arose from the (now largely discredited) theory that too much saturated fat was bad for health because it increased the LDL cholesterol content of the blood. We have seen above that Ancel Keys postulated the notion that saturated fat consumption led to heart disease due to the increase of LDL cholesterol it caused. We now know that cholesterol is largely formed in the body and that if you consume less cholesterol in your diet the body will create more to balance this. Your body actually needs cholesterol; it is vital for you to survive.

Cholesterol is a type of lipid that performs many essential jobs in the body including being the precursor to our sex hormones. Lipids are substances that don't dissolve in water or in blood. They travel through the bloodstream to reach different parts of the body. Every cell in the body has cholesterol as part of its structure and every cell in the body needs cholesterol to function. Forget about the myth of 'good' and 'bad' cholesterol.

It is true that some foods are high in cholesterol – eggs, red meat and organ meats like liver, for example. But it is now understood that eating a 'high cholesterol' diet has no effect on your body levels. Cholesterol is manufactured in the liver – if you ate a completely cholesterol-free diet your body would simply try to make more of this important nutrient.

There is also a serious consideration that excessively low levels of cholesterol (caused by medication with statins) may actually be one *cause* of dementia symptoms. (See the advice given by Dr Jerry Thomson in Chapter 4.) At least one researcher has suggested that low cholesterol levels are the *main* cause of dementia.[1]

Plant-based diets

Advice about eating a 'plant-based diet' is very fashionable at the moment and so successful has the media marketing been that many people are convinced that it is the only healthy diet. It is also marketed as a 'planet friendly' diet so that those adopting it can bask in the double warming glow of being both healthy and 'green'.

Up until recently someone who claimed to be eating a plant-based diet would probably be classed as 'vegan'. Vegans eat no animal product of any kind whereas vegetarians eschew meat but will eat eggs, milk, cheese and other animal products. In terms of health, there is a world of difference between the two diets. A vegetarian diet can be a completely healthy diet as all the nutrients the body requires can be obtained from vegetables and animal products combined even if no meat is eaten (we will discuss those who eat fish in addition – pescatarians – later).

Vegans maintain that their diet is also healthy, but the fact is that in a completely vegan diet some nutrients which are essential for human life are missing. These might include vitamin A (this can be obtained from beta-carotene, a vitamin A 'precursor', in plants but the conversion rate in the human body can be poor), vitamin B12, vitamin D3 and some trace elements such as taurine, zinc and iodine. Vitamin B12 is of particular interest because it plays an essential role in maintenance of the central nervous system and your body cannot manufacture it. You have to consume an average of 2.4 micrograms per day from food or supplements. There are no reliable plant sources of vitamin B12 apart from certain algae/seaweeds, but even here it is less 'bioavailable' to humans. It *is* found in a wide variety of animal-based foods. Most strict vegans will need to take a supplement of this vitamin. Symptoms of low levels of vitamin B12 can take a long while to surface and this means that many people when they start to adopt a vegan diet do not realise that they are becoming deficient.

A study in the journal *Neurology* in September 2008 found that brain volume loss was associated with the low levels of vitamin B12 often found in vegans and vegetarians. This study also found associations with Alzheimer's disease and other cognitive failures.[3]

Nowadays the popular 'plant-based diet' advice is more likely to suggest that we use plant-based foods (vegetables, fruit and beans and other pulses) as the major constituent of our diet and only include meat products as 'condiments' in very small amounts. The difficulty that arises with putting the plant-based diet advice into practice is that, in order to have a healthy diet whilst excluding (or dramatically reducing our intake of) certain classes of food, we need to be very aware of the nutritional quality of what we eat. It is important to combine different food elements to make sure that we get the right nutrients in the right quantities. Not many people have the knowledge or the time, or sometimes the sources of food, to do this with confidence.

There is also the question of misinformation. For example, many milk substitutes are available (oat mylk, soya mylk, almond mylk and so on) but, whilst these options give us something to add to our coffee if we do not want dairy milk, it is really important to know that none of them is actually 'milk' and none of them contains the same nutrients as milk. By calling these substitutes 'milk', the media may be causing people to think that they are using a like-for-like substitute with the same level of nutrition.

So, the biggest problem with plant-based diets is balancing the foods eaten to ensure an adequate intake of protein and certain vitamins and trace elements.

Interestingly for those of us who have begun to believe, due to the constant bombardment from the media, that eating red meat is bad for us, a new research paper suggests that there is little or no evidence to support this. Researchers from the Institute for Health Metrics and Evaluation (IHME) recently conducted a systematic review of published research to evaluate the relationships between unprocessed red meat consumption and six potential health outcomes including stroke, type 2 diabetes and colorectal cancer. They found no evidence that eating red meat increased the risk of stroke and only weak evidence of the effects on other health outcomes. They concluded: 'While there is some evidence that eating unprocessed red meat is associated with increased risk of disease incidence and mortality, it is weak and insufficient to make stronger or more conclusive recommendations.'[4]

Pescatarians

The pescatarian diet incorporates seafood (fish and aquatic animals) into an otherwise vegetarian diet. Pescatarians may or may not also consume animal products like eggs, cheese, milk and butter.

Fish, especially fatty fish like salmon, herring, and trout, are high in omega-3 fatty acids – fats that are essential to health and are involved in critical processes including regulating inflammation in the body. The body must get omega-3 fatty acids from food as it is unable to make it by itself. Fish contains the omega-3 fats eicosapentaenoic acid (EPA) and docosahexaenoic acid (DHA), which are also found in some animal-based foods (e.g. grass-fed beef) and algae.

Conversely, plant foods that provide omega-3 fats do so in the form alpha-linolenic acid (ALA), which is a precursor to EPA and DHA, and conversion of ALA to EPA and DHA in the human body is not very efficient. It relies on certain enzymes that may also be deficient.

Some research suggests that a good intake of certain vitamins and of DHA is a useful approach to delaying brain ageing and for protecting against the onset of Alzheimer's disease.[5]

One thing to keep in mind is that because a pescatarian diet includes a high amount of seafood, there may be a higher risk of exposure to certain toxic chemicals, including mercury, lead and polychlorinated biphenyls (PCB), that are known to accumulate in sea creatures.

The paleo diet

The principle behind the paleo diet is that it is what our Stone Age ancestors ate and therefore what millions of years of evolution adapted us for. While there can have been no single 'Stone Age' diet as what was eaten would have been determined by availability, it probably did not include cultivated foods, including particularly grain or dairy products. Proponents of the paleo diet believe that the human body has not evolved to process dairy, legumes and grains and that eating these foods could increase the risk of certain health conditions.

This diet can maintain good health if attention is paid to balancing the various constituents. However, the problem is that it is quite a difficult diet to maintain because it does exclude many straightforward and easily obtained foods, like bread, and most of us are used to including bread (how do you replace a simple sandwich for convenience?) and pasta in our diet and we are even encouraged to do so by 'standard' food advice. It can be a challenge to find suitable substitutes for these regular additions to meals. On the other hand, it is the processed carbohydrates which are most often condemned by nutritionists as unhealthy so excluding these from the diet would seem to be a healthy choice.

Gluten-free diet

Excluding gluten from the diet gained credence and popularity a few years ago, particularly after the mainstream nutritionists began to acknowledge that perhaps some people were 'sensitive' to gluten. Previously the line taken by the medical world was that there was a disease called coeliac disease; those who had this disease were genetically unable to process gluten and would need to follow a gluten-free diet for life. Coeliac disease was considered to be quite rare. In the UK, children are usually diagnosed when quite young and, once on a gluten-free diet, they thrive and can live normally.

It is now acknowledged that many more people have coeliac disease than was previously believed and often people are diagnosed as adults having suffered from various digestive symptoms all their life.

Gluten is a protein found in many grains, particularly wheat, and (for instance, in bread) gluten proteins form an elastic network that stretches and traps gas, allowing the bread to rise and retain moisture. This gives bread a softer and more acceptable texture. It is commonly postulated that modern wheat cultivation and bread manufacture results in a much higher gluten content in the bread we eat today and that this may be the reason that more people appear to be suffering from gluten sensitivity than in the past. Many people are convinced that they are sensitive to gluten, and the 'gluten-free diet' and gluten-free options in supermarkets and restaurants are now common. If you are gluten-sensitive, then it makes sense to follow a gluten-free diet. There is, however, no solid evidence at present that gluten of itself contributes to the risk of developing dementia.

Recommendations

There are many other special 'diets' that are pushed by the media, such as the keto diet the intermittent-fasting diet, the DASH diet and the Mediterranean diet. There is a wealth of literature which describes how people have cured themselves of diseases such as motor neurone disease, cancer and other devastating illnesses by radically changing what they eat, although usually they have used other interventions such as meditation, exercise and visualisation in addition. People who have cured themselves (the medical term used is 'gone into remission') are naturally enthusiastic about the radical diets they have adopted and frequently they have spread the word about these through social and more traditional media and some have become famous as living examples of the benefits of the diet they advocate. There is no denying that a change in diet has seemed to alter the course of their disease and in many cases effected a cure.

It can be very difficult to assess the benefits of some of the more radical diets since often they are so extreme that only the dedicated or desperate can find the will to follow them without fail. It does seem as though for some people a radical diet change has altered their health for the better. However, when we examine the many cases of disease cure through diet it becomes clear that these people were already ill, their immune systems were not functioning adequately and that only a radical change in their diet and habits could bring about improvement. It is hard to assess adequately the benefits of adopting dramatic changes in diet if you are generally well and are only considering the prevention of developing disease in the future. However, if you have warning signs like diabetes or AMD, then you might think about this approach in more depth.

The diet most highly recommended by the medical press is the Mediterranean diet. Our grandparents would probably recognise this diet as the 'good mixed diet' which was promulgated in their youth. While there is no single definition of this diet, it is typically high in vegetables, fruit, whole grains, beans, nuts and seeds, and olive oil, and includes fish and usually meat and dairy foods in limited quantities.

As far as dementia prevention is concerned, there are a few facts which we can follow and none of them requires dramatic changes to our diet or the seeking out of unusual 'health' foods or difficult food preparation. The key pointers to follow are reducing sugar/eliminating added sugar and avoiding ultra-processed foods.

Reduce sugar – eliminate added sugar

If you are confused by all the dietary advice and just want to do the simplest thing you can to reduce your chances of developing dementia, then cut sugar from your diet as much as possible. This is the most important factor with real evidence behind it.

When we refer to 'sugar' in the following paragraphs, what is meant is 'table sugar' – sucrose, which is made up of the two simple sugars glucose and fructose. However, bear in mind that fructose and glucose, which are often listed as ingredients on processed foods, are themselves sugars. Sugar is a very simple carbohydrate with no essential nutrients. It can make you gain weight, it causes excessive rises and dips in blood glucose level and it can cause type 2 diabetes (a major risk factor for dementia – see previous chapters). The trouble is that sugar is rather nice; it is a major constituent of so many foods and is added in smaller amounts to many more, so that we are not always aware that we are eating it.

One example of this is bread. If you make bread at home you will have to add a tiny amount of sugar to get the yeast started and, even if this were all that the bakers of mass-produced bread were doing, they would have to list 'sugar' as an ingredient because that is the law in UK. However, many versions of bread contain much larger amounts of added sugar and, if you compare various brands, some of them actually taste sweet because so much sugar has been added. Most of us would not consider that bread contained sugar. Sugar is also added to most breakfast cereals, even those considered healthy like muesli. 'Healthy' energy bars and cereal bars also contain added sugar.

Chapter 8

'Low fat' usually means more sugar

Most people who choose low-fat alternatives to everyday foods, such as dairy products, baked goods and ready-made dishes, do not realise that these foods are mostly higher in sugar content than the regular versions.[6] This is because the fat content is what gives much of the taste to food and if you reduce the fat content you have to 'up the taste', usually using sugar and/or salt.

If you take a random sample of foods in your store cupboard and carefully read the ingredients you are likely to be astonished at the things that contain sugar – for example, soy sauce, packet sauces, canned soup, baked beans and even gravy granules may all contain added sugar. It is almost impossible to avoid eating ANY sugar if you use any processed food at all.

However, you can do a great deal to reduce the amount of sugar you consume without major inconvenience. Firstly, do not add sugar to drinks. It is easy to become someone who 'does not take sugar' in hot drinks by simply reducing the amount you add very slowly (perhaps by half a teaspoon) until you no longer need the taste. Secondly, avoid packet breakfast cereals unless they contain no added sugar. Read the label of your favourite cereal carefully – even 'healthy' whole grain, high-fibre cereals, and this includes most muesli, may contain added sugar. Next, if you eat bread, start to read the list of ingredients and switch to a version with no added sugar.

You can follow this routine with all the common foods that you eat. After a while it becomes a habit to peruse the label and you will find you become quite clever at spotting sugar in all its forms (sucrose, fructose, glucose and anything ending in 'ose' or 'ol' etc). You can very often find an alternative version of sauces, soups and tinned foods which do not contain added sugar.

If you do not like the taste of the alternative, consider whether this is because it is less sweet; then you may begin to see your whole diet in a different light.

It is also true that, as you consume less sugar, you will find yourself wanting sugar less. This is because it is an addictive substance (particularly when combined with fats as in cream cakes and chocolate), and the more you eat the more you crave. Once your diet is low in sugar you are likely to find the odd cake or biscuit too sweet and possibly be unable to finish it.

Of course, no one wants to do without any pleasures in their diet and it is a fact that cakes, biscuits and ice cream can be an enjoyable treat; how sad our life would be without treats. If you are an ardent 'anti-sugar' missionary, you may also find that you are less welcome as a guest. So, the answer is to treat sugar and sweet foods as 'treats' to be eaten occasionally – without guilt – and enjoyed because you eat them rarely.

Eat less processed and ultra-processed food

The definition of 'ultra-processed' food is long and complicated but Dr Chris Van Tulleken in his book *Ultra Processed People: Why Do We All Eat Stuff That Isn't Food...and Why can't We Stop* suggests that any foodstuff that contains ingredients you don't have in your kitchen is an indicator that it is an ultra-processed food.[7]

A great deal of the food we eat is processed – even cooking vegetables involves processing them – but ultra-processed foods (UPF) are foods that have gone through industrial processes like refining, bleaching and hydrogenating and are then combined with additives and assembled using industrial techniques. You may believe that you never consume such foods but a glance at the label of your favourite cereal may convince you otherwise.

As an adjunct to cutting sugar you may like to consider reducing processed carbohydrates in your everyday diet. These include items like white flour, pastry (except pastry made at home with wholemeal flour) packet and canned foods and 'ready meals'. Once again, if you begin reading labels and lists of ingredients on cans and packets, you may find yourself amazed at the additional items which have been added to the main food. Often these are such things as stabilisers or preservatives which have been added to prolong the shelf-life of food and, as such, are not intrinsically bad in themselves. The concern is that the continual consumption of these additives which are not naturally found in food may cause an accumulation in the body of alien substances. In many cases we do not know what damage this may cause to the human body.

How do we reduce consumption of processed foods? It is quite simple. Make every effort to cook from scratch and reduce to a minimum the use of packet, tinned and ready-made foods. It can seem very time consuming at first but you can quickly get into a routine of making batches of soups or stews or casseroles which can be frozen for later use. If you do not have a freezer you can still cook enough of a basic recipe to make two or more meals and refrigerate the leftovers for the next day. Once you begin to read the lists of ingredients you will probably be amazed at how simple it can be to make most dishes at home and it is frequently no more expensive than to buy them ready made. They often taste better too.

The exception is food items like sausages which are complicated to make and require special equipment. Once again, here the answer is to read labels and choose the product which has the least number of additional ingredients. There are specialist suppliers like farm shops and butchers who sell high-quality less-processed foods, but they are likely to be more expensive and most of us have to tread a fine line between thinking of our future health and thinking of our budget.

Conclusion

Actions to take now include:
- Stop adding sugar to drinks.

- Do not buy soft drinks or flavoured water (these all contain sugar).
- Reduce intake of cakes, biscuits and pastries to a minimum.
- Read food labels and choose to buy foods that are low in sugar (or sugar-free) and have relatively few ingredients.
- Cook dishes from scratch where possible and don't add white flour products to your cooking.

Chapter 9

Exercise for body and brain

Key points:
- Physical exercise of any type including walking and gardening is beneficial for the brain.
- Physical exercise benefits the cardiovascular system, reducing the risk of vascular dementia.
- It also seems to be protective against all types of dementia, especially in women.
- Exercising the brain builds cognitive reserve.
- To 'exercise your brain', constantly try new activities, meet new people, explore new places and learn new things.
- It is never too late to start exercising.

Exercise for the body

There is a large body of evidence which suggests that physical exercise not only prevents the development of dementia but also slows the rate of decline in people who are already diagnosed with symptoms of dementia.

We are all familiar with the constantly reiterated mantra that 'exercise is good for you' and most of us take this for granted.

However, perhaps we should examine why exercise is considered to be a good thing and especially why physical exercise is said to be of such benefit to the brain.

Most advice on exercising gives greater emphasis to the benefits to the cardiovascular system but it goes much further than that. One medical internet site (NHS Choices) suggests that the health benefits of regular exercise include:

- up to a 35% lower risk of coronary heart disease and stroke.
- up to a 50% lower risk of type 2 diabetes.
- up to a 50% lower risk of colon cancer.
- up to a 20% lower risk of breast cancer.
- a 30% lower risk of early death.
- up to an 83% lower risk of osteoarthritis.
- up to a 68% lower risk of hip fracture.
- a 30% lower risk of falls (among older adults).
- up to a 30% lower risk of depression... as well as a 30% lower risk of dementia.[1]

Exercise is known to have multiple positive effects in older adults, including those with disabilities. In particular, exercise prevents and reduces the risk of developing secondary conditions that arise from functional decline and lack of physical use.

Physical exercise is a considered to be a primary and secondary preventer of cardiovascular illness, particularly that due to ischaemic heart disease (blocked coronary arteries). Regular physical exercise is thought to implement its beneficial effects through: reducing the incidence and severity of obesity and the consequent risk of type 2 diabetes ; improving glucose tolerance; preventing the development of blood clots; and lowering blood pressure. (Glucose tolerance and the part played in the risk of dementia by diabetes has been discussed in other chapters.)

It is thought that low physical activity roughly doubles the risk of coronary heart disease and is a major risk factor for stroke. As well as the direct physical benefits on the body's cardiovascular and metabolic parameters, exercise also provides benefits through reducing the effects of stress, ameliorating and preventing depressive illness and anxiety in those who are at risk of, or suffering from, cardiovascular disease, and through improvements in self-esteem.

Physical exercise and vascular dementia

The evidence that physical exercise has a beneficial effect on the cardiovascular system is now considered incontrovertible. A healthy cardiovascular system helps to protect against the development of vascular dementia. Vascular dementia, as previously explained, is caused by problems in the supply of blood to the brain. Typically, the symptoms of this type of dementia begin suddenly, sometimes following a stroke. Vascular dementia also tends to follow a 'stepped' progression, with symptoms remaining at a constant level for a time and then suddenly deteriorating. Sometimes no precipitating stroke is recognised but when a history is taken, carers can recall a time or an incident from which symptoms seemed to stem. Often the cause is a so-called 'mini-stroke' (a transient ischaemic attack or TIA for short).

Occasionally carers will not be able to pinpoint a precipitating event and will maintain that the loss of cognition has happened slowly and almost imperceptibly. In such cases it seems that there has been a very slow and gradual reduction in supply of blood to the brain, perhaps by small blood vessels becoming blocked, and it is the cumulative effects of this reduction of blood supply which causes the cognitive losses affecting memory and the ability to carry out actions of everyday living.

To be healthy and function properly, brain cells need a good supply of blood. Blood is delivered through a network of blood vessels called the vascular system. If the vascular system within the brain becomes damaged (for example, by a stroke or trauma) and blood cannot reach the brain cells, the cells will eventually die. This may lead to the onset of vascular dementia. It is now believed that vascular 'events' may also have a bearing on the development of Alzheimer's disease.

It follows that, since exercise has a beneficial effect on the cardiovascular system as a whole, it will have this effect on the part of the vascular system that supplies blood to the brain. A better supply of blood to the brain will prevent or decrease damage to the brain and the manifestation of that damage by symptoms of dementia.

Physical exercise and improved cognition

Vascular disease is not, however, the whole story and in actual fact the mechanism by which physical activity improves cognition in older people (at least in those at risk of dementia) is not completely clear. Nevertheless, the results of a significant body of research do seem to demonstrate that physical activity is a key to the non-development of dementia symptoms.

SJ Colcombe and colleagues, in a study to look at the relationship between aerobic fitness and brain volume, observed 59 healthy but sedentary volunteers, aged 60-79 years, who were living in the community (i.e. not in residential care homes).[2] Half of the group undertook aerobic training whilst the other half participated in a toning and stretching 'control' group. Significant increases in brain volume, in both grey and white matter regions, were found after six months' trial in those who participated in the aerobic fitness training but not in those who had been taking part in the stretching and toning (non-aerobic) control group. Along with other research, this study suggests that the scope of beneficial effects of aerobic exercise extend beyond just cardiovascular health, and that there is a direct effect upon brain health and volume.

Danielle Laurin and colleagues in a study coordinated through the University of Ottawa and the Division of Aging and Seniors, Health Canada, set out to explore the association between physical activity and the risk of cognitive impairment and dementia. Their research showed that, compared with no exercise, physical activity was associated with 'lower risks ....of dementia of any type'.[3] This study of a large number of people emphasised that significant trends for increased protection (against dementia) were observed with greater physical activity and this possibly protective effect was particularly noticeable in women.

One theory is that exercise has an effect on brain plasticity (see below). Carl W Cotman and Nicole C Berchtold suggested the possibility that exercise acted directly on the molecular structure of the brain itself and that beneficial effects were not simply connected with a general benefit to overall health. In an animal study using rats and mice given the opportunity (but not forced) to use an exercise wheel, Cotman and Berchtold focused on a substance called brain-derived neurotrophic factor (BDNF) because this factor makes possible neuronal connectivity. In simple words, this factor allows neurons to connect to one another and change their connections when new skills are being learned. The researchers expected that the response to exercise would be restricted to motor sensory systems of the brain such as the cerebellum, primary cortical areas or basal ganglia. Amazingly, after several days of voluntary wheel-running, they found increased levels of BDNF in the hippocampus, a part of the brain normally associated with higher cognitive function.[4]

The hippocampus has important roles in the consolidation of information from short-term memory to long-term memory and in spatial navigation. In Alzheimer's disease, the hippocampus is one of the first regions of the brain to suffer damage. Memory problems and disorientation appear among the first symptoms of the disease. This research indicated that exercise actually strengthens the neural structure, helping the neurones to make connections with each other.[4]

So, it appears that even a little light exercise is better than no exercise at all for our cognitive function. The next question might be 'is there more improvement in cognition the more exercise you undertake?'. One large-scale US study – part of the National Long Term Care Survey – in which levels of exercise and cognitive impairment status were measured over a 10-year period was particularly interesting in this respect. The results showed not only that exercise had a beneficial effect on cognition but that the number and different types of exercise performed were inversely associated with the onset of cognitive improvement. The interesting point is that whilst exercise of any kind was found to be beneficial, the number of different types of exercise made a difference. Those engaging in four different types of exercise over a two-week period decreased their risk (of cognitive impairment) when compared with those who engaged in one type of exercise only.[5] It isn't clear why more and different types of exercise seem more beneficial. It is possible that taking part in a greater variety of exercise means that people get more social and cognitive stimulation in addition to the beneficial effect of exercise upon the brain. It may also be connected with multiple activity input to the brain increasing plasticity (see page 15).

'Exercise' in this context does not mean necessarily sweating it out in a gym. The study took account of all types of exercise even walking and gardening or 'yard work'.

A study involving Swedish twins investigated whether exercise earlier in life had an effect on the probability of developing dementia at a later stage of life. Scientists like to use twins in their research due to their genotypes and family environments tending to be similar. In this research, scientists were investigating whether those who exercised in mid-life (well before any signs of dementia might manifest) were less likely to become demented later in life. In this case the researchers concluded that 'light exercise such as gardening or walking and regular exercise involving sports were associated with reduced odds of dementia compared to hardly any exercise'.[6]

David Snowdon in his book *Aging With Grace*, an account of the well-known 'Nun's Study' (see Chapter 1) relates the story of a conversation with Sister Nicolette (then aged 91) in which he asks her to what she attributes her good health and longevity. She replies that she has an exercise programme which involves walking several miles a day. When asked when she started this programme, Sister Nicolette replies, 'When I was 70'.[7] So perhaps we might query when 'mid-life' begins.

Many researchers point out that the 'exercise effect' may not be necessarily as clear cut as it appears. It could be that people who exercise more tend to lead healthier lives generally, eating a healthy diet, avoiding smoking and keeping to a moderate alcohol intake for example. Nevertheless, the fact remains, that those who exercise more have a lower risk of developing dementia in later life.

Physical exercise when there are early signs of dementia

Exercise is beneficial even after memory problems have manifested themselves. There are a number of studies which link Alzheimer's disease and other dementias with a more general physical deterioration. People with dementia are more likely to show signs of under-nutrition, to have a higher risk of falls (and consequent fractures) and a more rapid decline in mobility. Improving the physical condition of people with dementia may therefore extend their independent mobility and their quality of life. Even quite elderly people can improve their cardiovascular function, their ability to move muscle groups easily and without pain, their balance and their strength, with a systematic exercise programme. Improved flexibility and balance are likely to reduce the possibility of falls which may result in injury or admission to hospital. If you read Chapter 10 on 'Avoiding confounding factors' you will realise that it is important to avoid injury and admission to hospital where at all possible. So, an exercise programme is worth undertaking to improve the general health and wellbeing of anyone with the beginnings of dementia. Further than this, a number of studies have been carried out which look specifically at exercise induced benefits in cognitive functioning in people with dementia.

Exercise is known to have a good effect on cardiorespiratory fitness. A study in 2009 examined the relationship between cardiorespiratory fitness and regional brain volume in a sample of people with early Alzheimer's disease (AD) to non-demented controls. In this study, those in early-stage AD with a higher level of cardiorespiratory fitness had a higher temporal lobe volume, particularly in the areas associated with executive processing. These parts of the brain are affected early in AD. This seemed to apply to people carrying the ApoE4 gene as much as to those who did not.[8] (See Chapters 1 and 6 for discussion of ApoE4.)

There have been other studies to examine whether exercise programmes will improve memory in those with early-stage dementia. A physical activity intervention trial was conducted in which participants who reported memory problems were encouraged to undertake 150 minutes per week of physical activity of moderate intensity.[9] Participants were tested at the start of the trial and after six, 12 and 18 months to see if their cognitive function improved. This trial showed that exercise improved cognitive function in older adults with memory problems. The improvement was apparent after six months and persisted for 12 months after discontinuation of the trial. The results showed that participants who undertook the exercise did better on a standard Alzheimer's disease test (ADAS-Cog) and had a better delayed recall than those who were allocated to a control 'usual care' group. In this trial the usual choice of exercise by participants was walking. A few people chose to include some light strength-training as well.

A 2009 study which tested the effects of a combined diet and exercise intervention in people at risk of developing Alzheimer's Disease included 1800 people, 1598 of whom showed no signs of dementia at the start of the study. This study used a valuation of 1.3 hours per week of vigorous activity (aerobic dancing, jogging, playing handball), 2.4 hours of moderate exercise (cycling, swimming, hiking or playing tennis) and 4 hours of light exercise (walking, playing golf, bowling, gardening). Even this relatively small amount of physical activity was associated with a reduction in the risk for developing Alzheimer's Disease.[10]

Patricia Heyn and colleagues conducted a meta-analysis of research on exercise and dementia. A meta-analysis, as described in earlier chapters, is a method of contrasting and combining results from different studies in the hope of identifying patterns among study results. This paper looked at a number of randomised trials with participants over 65 year of age. The meta-analysis concluded that exercise training increased fitness, physical function, cognitive function, and positive behaviour in people with dementia and related cognitive impairments.[11] The authors of this paper also mentioned the problem of motivating people with dementia to exercise and of the possible need to adjust exercise programmes for dementia needs (see below, page 152).

Physical exercise with mild cognitive impairment (MCI)

MCI may be an indicator of later dementia. Laura Baker conducted a study which looked at the effects of aerobic exercise on cognition in older adults with this diagnosis. This was a six-month randomised controlled clinical trial, although it included only a small number (33) of participants. Participants undertook either high-intensity aerobic exercise or, in the case of the control group, supervised stretching exercises. The study concluded that physical exercise had an effect on cognition, glucose metabolism and cardiac fitness. Again, (as in the Lauren study) this effect was particularly noticeable in women.[12]

Physical exercise with dementia

A randomised controlled trial by Linda Teri and colleagues reported in a 2003 paper investigated the effect of exercise plus a behavioural management programme given to carers of people with dementia. The exercise component of the programme included aerobic/endurance activities, strength-training, balance and flexibility training and carers were trained to instigate and supervise this exercise programme at home. In addition to the exercise programme, carers were educated about dementia and its effects and to increase physical and social activity. After three months on the programme there were definite improvements in physical functioning and significantly, improvements in the level of depression in those with dementia who had been randomly assigned to the programme compared to the 'control' group.[13] As described in Chapter 1, depression often accompanies dementia and is an added difficulty both for those with this combined diagnosis and for those who are caring for them.

A further study conducted from 1993 to 2003 (so over a long period) examined whether participation in physical activity reduced the rate of cognitive decline after accounting for participation in cognitively stimulating activities. Initially results showed that more hours of activity were associated with a slower rate of decline in cognitive function. However, when results were adjusted to allow for the effect of cognitively stimulating activity it was felt that the effect of physical activity was not significant.[13a]

Although this study seems at first sight to negate some other research which shows the positive effects of physical exercise, it is not as clear cut as that. Participants in the study who exercised regularly showed a slower rate of cognitive decline. What is clear is that those people who took part in regular exercise more often probably also took part in cognitively stimulating activities as well. In actual fact, physical activity is in itself cognitively stimulating and generally exercising more results also in a more full and varied social life. For example, walking might involve going to new places, meeting others during the walk and conversation in the course of the walk.

Physical exercise and cognition: Conclusions

The evidence is clear even if we do not yet understand entirely why exercise makes a positive difference. People who exercise are less likely to develop dementia and this seems especially to apply to women. Light exercise is better than no exercise at all.

It is clear, too, that it is never too late to begin exercising. Those who already have signs of dementia or who have MCI can still obtain benefit from commencing an exercise programme. Exercise, it seems, is a wonderful prophylactic and a treatment, and it is free.

What more could you ask for?

Exercise for the brain

'But,' people ask me, 'isn't it important to "exercise the brain"?' Most people equate brain exercise with things like doing puzzles, crosswords and word games. These activities certainly do 'exercise the brain' but there is no hard evidence that such activities make one less likely to develop dementia. To consider this further we have to go back to what was said in Chapter 1 about **cognitive reserve**.

The idea of a 'reserve' in the brain comes from the observation scientists have made from post-mortem examinations that some people whose brains had extensive Alzheimer's disease pathology, clinically had no or very little manifestation of the disease. Reserve is perceived as having both passive and active components. Passive components are structural features involving the anatomy of the brain. Active reserve is taken to mean the efficiency of the neural networks and the brain's ability to compensate or use alternative networks after an injury such as, for example, a stroke. Doctor Yaakov Stern in his paper 'Cognitive reserve in ageing and Alzheimer's disease', suggests similarly that the concept of cognitive reserve may take two forms. In 'neural reserve' the existing brain networks are more efficient or have a greater capacity to resist damage. In 'neural compensation', other brain networks may compensate for the networks that are damaged.

Cognitive reserve then is the ability of the brain either to resist damage or to compensate for damage that has occurred. Stern suggests that: 'lifelong experiences, including educational and occupational attainment, and leisure activities in later life, can increase this reserve.'[14]

What we are talking about here is experiences, education and activities which enable our brain to stimulate neural pathways and expand. Word games and puzzles might expand the brain if we have never before attempted them, but if we are continually working at activities with which we are familiar all we are doing is reinforcing the pathways in the brain which are already formed. We could liken this to a field of grass. If someone walks through the grass in a certain direction they may leave a faint path. If others follow the same path, it becomes more pronounced. Since the human tendency is to take the way of least resistance, others may walk the same path and make a more obvious track. The track becomes a beaten footpath and eventually it becomes 'the way' to cross the field. The brain works in the same way. If we enjoy a certain type of puzzle and practise it often, the brain becomes very proficient at doing that type of puzzle. This will not however help the brain to stretch itself and become better *in general*.

The best way to 'exercise the brain' is to constantly try new activities, meet new people, explore new places and learn new things. There is nothing to stop anyone doing this as they grow older. It may sometimes seem more difficult to learn new things or seem to take longer, but no matter what age you are you can do it. Taking up a new language, reading a different book from your usual choice, learning to play a musical instrument, joining a new club, trying a new activity – all these things are real 'brain exercise' and are likely to help to keep dementia at bay.

If this seems difficult then think about taking small steps to work towards this. You could begin by just doing some everyday things in a different way. Here are some examples:

- Use a different supermarket for your weekly shop.
- Take a different route when you go for a walk.
- Use a different garage to refuel your car.
- Read a different daily newspaper.
- Try a new recipe for your main meal.

You may be surprised to find that doing some of these things makes you slightly uncomfortable – you are getting out of your 'comfort zone' and this is a really good thing from the point of view of your brain. You may find that you enjoy a different route, different food, an unfamiliar shop. These are small steps which will fire different neurones in the brain and prepare the way for new neural pathways to develop.

But don't stop there! Having prepared the way and got yourself used to doing things a little differently, think about some bigger steps – perhaps you could take a journey to visit a place which you have been thinking was too distant or too complicated to arrange. Or you might consider visiting an exhibition you would not normally choose to see or watching a film that you thought was not quite to your taste. Sometimes going 'out on a limb' like this can lead to a completely fresh outlook on life and a new interest. At the worst you will have caused your brain to make an effort and experienced something different.

You may think that you are too old to learn something new such as playing a musical instrument or speaking a different language, but research shows differently. Shirley Leanos and her colleagues conducted a study to find out whether learning multiple real-world skills simultaneously is possible in older adults and whether it helped to improve their cognitive abilities. They found that learning multiple skills simultaneously increased cognitive abilities in older adults to levels similar to performance of people who were several years younger.[15]

You might consider achieving two things at once – improving your physical exercise levels and learning a new skill by taking up a new sport or active hobby. Many forms of physical exercise are particularly suitable for older people such as gardening, bowls and golf, and for those who enjoyed team games in the past, there are now many adaptations such as 'walking football' and 'walking netball' available.[16]

Conclusion

There is ample evidence to show that physical exercise has an effect in the prevention of dementia. When we talk about brain exercise we have to think beyond puzzles and word games and really extend the mind by attempting new activities and continued learning however old we are.

Key things to do include:

- Assess how much physical exercise you presently do.
- Consider what other exercise you could fit into your schedule.

- Investigate enjoyable ways to increase your exercise level.
- Get outside of your 'comfort zone' regularly.
- Don't accept that you are 'too old to learn' new things.

Chapter 10

Modifiable risk factors

Alcohol, air pollution, smoking and vaping, infections, falls, hospitalisation, surgery, EMFs and hearing loss

Risk factors for dementia that we can modify include:
- Alcohol consumption
- Air pollution
- Smoking
- Infections
- Falls
- Hospital admissions
- Electromagnetic frequencies (EMFs)
- Hearing loss.

In this chapter, we will be looking at what are described as 'modifiable risk factors for dementia'. This means factors that can be reduced by changes to lifestyle or specific precautions. Risks have to be weighed up when decisions are taken – for example, having certain types of surgical procedure may raise the risk of developing dementia but choosing not to have the procedure may be a risk to life. In these cases, there may be steps that can be taken to reduce the dementia risk and these will be discussed.

Alcohol consumption

The *Lancet Report* (see Chapter 1) lists a reduction in alcohol consumption as one of the modifiable risk factors for dementia, suggesting that this is one lifestyle area where each individual can take steps to reduce their risk.[1] In Chapter 3, alcohol-related dementia has been extensively discussed and so what we will look at here is the possibility of regular social drinking affecting the risk of developing dementia.

There are important limitations when we consider research on alcohol consumption. Most research relies on self-reporting which is known to be unreliable and there has been little research on assessing the effect of alcohol consumption over a lifetime. Nor are the research conclusions necessarily clear. A 23-year follow-up to the Whitehall 11 cohort study published in the *British Medical Journal* in 2018 concluded that: 'The risk of dementia was increased in people who abstained from alcohol in midlife or consumed more than 14 units/week', suggesting that not drinking at all carries the same risk as drinking too much.[2]

There are other health risks connected to excessive drinking and so you might consider that moderate social drinking is the best option if you want to avoid dementia.

Air pollution

Research is not yet conclusive about the link between air pollution and dementia but it is highly suggestive that the link exists. Unfortunately, research does not yet pinpoint which pollutants might raise the risk the most. Some research papers have examined the connection between particulate matter (pm) and dementia. In particular, two papers reported on research into pm from wood-burning stoves and traffic-related air pollution in Sweden and concluded that pollution from wood-burning stoves and traffic might be important risk factors.[3, 4]

A study to investigate whether the incidence of dementia is related to residential levels of air and noise pollution in London was published in 2018 and concluded that there was evidence of a positive association between residential levels of air pollution across London and being diagnosed with dementia.[5]

These are quite frightening conclusions, although managing the risk of dementia in connection with air pollution is difficult. If you live in an area of high pollution you might want to consider moving house. Unfortunately, there is no guarantee that pollution levels in any area are likely to remain the same given the extent of road development and the extensive residential building in many areas.

You could of course take precautions by only going outside when traffic volumes are low, not using solid fuel for heating, and avoiding the use of candles and tea-lights indoors. There is also some evidence of air pollution from chemicals used in cleaning products and you might choose to avoid these where possible. Some people might choose to wear a mask when walking in an area of high traffic pollution.

This is a risk area which is difficult to assess and also difficult to address in terms of modifying one's lifestyle.

Smoking

This is a simple one as addressed in more detail on page 45. Smoking is bad for your health generally and, although some of the direct research about smoking and dementia is not necessarily conclusive, the damage that smoking does to your general health is now considered to be irrefutable. For example, smoking increases the possibility of stroke or vascular disease both of which are risk factors for dementia. If you are a smoker, then you can reduce your risk of developing dementia by stopping the habit.

Vaping (using e-cigarettes)

The safety and long-term health effects of using e-cigarettes or other vaping products are still not well known but preliminary research suggests vaping poses risks to heart health as well the dangers involved in inhaling chemicals.

In a 2019 review the authors point out that e-liquid aerosols contain particulates, oxidising agents, aldehydes and nicotine. inhaled, these aerosols are likely to affect the heart and circulatory system.

It also needs to be remembered that people vape to inhale nicotine (in many cases, in an effort to wean themselves off cigarette smoking) and nicotine is a harmful substance.[6]

Infections

There are some interesting ideas around dementia (and in particular Alzheimer's disease) being the result of infection. This is a different hypothesis from the suggestion that infections can result in dementia (see below).

There are also diseases which are known to be associated with dementia – for example, Huntingdon's disease, motor neurone disease and, in some cases, AIDS. However, if you have one of these diseases you will already know about the risk of dementia symptoms. What we are concerned with in this chapter is the dementia symptoms that can result after an unrelated infection. I am frequently meeting clients who say (and whose nearest relatives agree) that they were functioning well cognitively until they were ill (with Covid, 'flu, a chest infection or other seemingly unrelated illness) and whose dementia symptoms seemed to stem from that infection. It is not always possible to determine whether the illness brought the symptoms to the fore or whether the infection was the cause. Sometimes I advise a client to take time to convalesce from their illness before assuming that they have dementia and when I worked in the diagnostic memory clinic, the consultant psychiatrist would not make a diagnosis until any infection or delirium caused by an infection had been recovered from. Frequently people are diagnosed in hospital when they have been admitted for an infection and one cannot but be concerned as to whether the lingering effects of the infection were to blame for the loss of cognition.

Without suggesting that you become obsessed with your health, it is worth emphasising that you should take even minor infections more seriously as you age. Generally, older people are retired from paid employment so if that describes you, make use of this leisure time to take things more slowly if you have a minor illness and give yourself plenty of time to recover. Do not try to 'work through' any illness but do all you can in the way of early nights, good nutrition and refusing extra commitments to recover your full strength.

Falls

It was once suggested to me that you can tell if you are considered to be old if someone says you have 'had a fall'. Younger people fall over but older people 'have a fall'.

Children and elderly people are both prone to falls but whereas children usually get up and carry on after falling (perhaps with some interim crying) and frequently show no long-term ill effects, elderly people are usually less able to get up without help and are more likely to injure themselves when they fall. There are many causes of falls in the elderly, including poor balance, postural hypotension (low blood pressure when standing up), failing eyesight, failure to pick the feet up sufficiently when walking and difficulty grabbing handrails or grab bars.

Falls can be a major cause of increasing frailty as we get older. In the first place, any injuries as a result of falling will take longer to heal. Brittle bones may mean a broken hip or wrist (two common injuries in the elderly) and this may mean a hospital stay with all the accompanying problems (see below). Broken bones and other injuries, such as sprains, may also result in less mobility which will affect any exercise programme.

The other very real evil is the loss of confidence which comes after a fall. Even just one fall can mean that you become more fearful about walking over rough ground or negotiating steps. And every time you avoid a possible obstacle 'in case you might fall' the loss of confidence increases – you may even get 'flashbacks' where you picture the fall in your mind and get agitated.

You may think that as falling over is accidental there is little you can do about this compounding factor. Of course accidents happen and we cannot necessarily prevent them, but we can take steps to mitigate the risk of falls. One very important step is to have regular eyesight checks and to wear your visual aids (such as spectacles) if you need to do so. Many elderly people have difficulty with peripheral vision and your optometrist can discuss this and any remedies or precautions with you. If you are diabetic or have an eye problem such as glaucoma, then be sure to have your vision checked regularly. Take care also to watch where you are going and not to be distracted when walking over unfamiliar or rough ground.

Exercise is very good at reducing the risk of falls. It helps you to improve your balance and to adjust your activity to suit your ability. It strengthens the limbs and encourages flexibility. So all the advice in Chapter 9 will also help you to avoid a severe fall.

You should also make any sensible adjustments to your environment. In the house, make sure that there are no loose rugs, or items lying around to make trip hazards. When reaching into high places, use properly adjusted steps and step stools or ask someone younger to reach down items you need. Lighting is very important and I am often worried that my clients may be carried away by media suggestions about reducing lighting to 'save the planet' when they should be increasing the light in their home to save their physical health. In particular, I advise the use of full-spectrum daylight bulbs in living areas during the winter and after dark.

In the garden, have any loose paving attended to, get handrails fitted if necessary, sweep up wet leaves and don't attempt gardening tasks which may carry the risk of falling.

When out and about, be aware of your environment and be careful not to be distracted when crossing roads, climbing steps and negotiating unfamiliar places.

Injuries, hospital admission and loss of confidence can all contribute to the development of dementia and doing your best to avoid inadvertent falls will mitigate this risk factor.

Hospital admissions

A stay in hospital can often be the result of a fall with the attendant injury or of an infection which is not caught in time to be treated at home. People often used to say casually on hearing that someone was admitted to hospital, 'Well, they are in the best place', but for people who have dementia this may not always be true. Hospitals are confusing places and if you are already confused, a stay in hospital is likely to make your confusion worse. The environment is strange, there are numerous unknown people coming and going, you may be moved frequently between wards and if you are also in pain or feeling unwell it all adds up to a bad experience. To make matters worse, it is sometimes the case that visitors are discouraged – especially if there is any infection involved.

Hospitalisation can in itself lead to functional decline so a prolonged stay in hospital is really best avoided.[7]

Of course, a hospital stay is sometimes the only answer to the situation where emergencies are concerned and carers should not compromise their own health and the wellbeing of their loved one by insisting that they can manage at home if this is not the case. If you can manage at home or you can organise some extra help, then by all means make sure the hospital stay is as short as possible. In this you may be aided by the hospital who will want to avoid having any 'bed-blockers', but you may also be hindered by social care teams who have a responsibility to ensure that people discharged from hospital will be able to cope and be looked after adequately.

Sometimes social care can be helpful and you may be able to benefit from some interim care help from visiting care workers. Many of my clients have found this made all the difference after hospital discharge and, in some cases, it has led them to arrange longer-term home-care which improved their quality of life.

Hospitalisation with dementia

If you are caring for someone with dementia and a hospital stay is inevitable due to an injury or infection, then there are things you can do to help. Firstly, try to visit as much as possible. The last couple of years have made things difficult in this regard but in normal times most hospital ward staff will be only too glad if you can come in to help your cared-for, especially at busy times like meal times (and especially if your cared-for needs encouragement to eat). Your presence as a familiar face will be most reassuring to your cared-for and you will be able to tell staff about certain things which may be important.

You can also do your best to make sure that nursing staff know about your cared-for's dementia. The Alzheimer's Society in the UK produce a very useful document called 'This is Me' which you can complete on behalf of your cared-for and send into hospital with them. It explains many simple things like the name preferred, any likes/dislikes/allergies and any important points (for example, a fear of needles or other things) which will be helpful for hospital staff to know. It is an excellent initiative but it does rely on hospital staff actually reading it.

When your loved one is discharged from hospital expect some difficulties. They are likely to be more confused for a few weeks as well as upset by the change in environment. You might think that they will be glad to be home but, because of their memory problems, home may seem strange at first and they may have forgotten home routines. Any extra help you can get will benefit you, but the person with dementia may not find strange carers coming into the home a good thing from their point of view.

Try to be patient – usually things will settle down with time, but often a hospital stay does seem to make dementia symptoms worse, which is why it is to be avoided if possible.

Elective surgery

This brings us on to a related topic. We are used to the notion that many physical problems can be improved with surgery – cataracts, hip and knee replacement and hernia repairs are just some of the common surgical procedures often performed on older people. For many of us these surgical procedures are a great boon. Being able to see clearly again or being without the severe pain of an arthritic hip or knee can give a new lease of life. However, even for someone who does not have dementia these surgical procedures are not without risk – a risk that will be explained to you beforehand and which both you and the surgeon concerned will want to consider carefully.

Some very new research has highlighted the discovery of a brain membrane (the subarachnoid lymphatic-like membrane or SLYM) which encases the brain and keeps separate cerebrospinal fluid that contains waste products from 'fresh' cerebrospinal fluid. Researchers believe that damage to the SLYM could play a part in the development of of neurodegenerative diseases such as dementia. At the time of writing it is being postulated that the SLYM could be damaged by certain surgical procedures such as lumbar punctures. This is new research information so not enough is known about this possibility at present.[8]

Anaesthetic delirium is not dementia, although it has similar (but short-lived) symptoms (see page 36).

Electro-magnetic frequencies (EMF)

Electronic smog (or e-smog) is the accumulation of electronic fields. These are emitted from all sorts of electrical appliances: wiring, mobile phones and satellite-based communications, for example. Of particular concern are cordless phone bases, wi-fi routers, mobile phones and computers.

This is a potentially controversial area of investigation since most governments refuse to acknowledge any possible effects on humans of radio frequencies. However, there have been some research papers which have raised concerns.

A great deal of attention has been focused on the effect of mobile phone masts on birds and bees. It has been postulated that birds have been diverted from their normal migratory paths and that bees have been confused by radio frequencies.

Robert Beason and Peter Semm drew attention to the effects of a radio frequency signal similar to the signal produced by global systems for mobile telephone networks on neurones of the avian brain and found that such stimulation resulted in changes in the amount of neural activity by more than half of the brain cells.[9]

A few scientists have expressed similar concerns about the effects of radio frequencies on humans. Andrew Miller and colleagues highlighted the detrimental effects of radio frequency radiation particularly in connection with mobile (cell) phones and concluded that the International Agency for Research on Cancer (IRAC) and the World Health Organization (WHO) ought to complete a systematic review of the health effects. This paper also suggested that their conclusions gave justification for governments, public health authorities and physicians/allied health professionals to warn the population that having a cell phone next to the body is harmful, and to support measures to reduce all exposures to radio frequency radiation.[10]

Andrew Goldsworthy, a scientific adviser to Electrosensitivity UK, has written a very easy-to-understand explanation of how the biological effects of weak electromagnetic fields can cause damage to human cells resulting in many effects, including dementia.[11]

Protecting yourself from the effects of radio frequency radiation or electromagnetic smog can appear almost impossible given the ubiquity of mobile phones, electric appliances and wi-fi equipment. Our world is now an 'electronic world' and it is not easy to avoid being exposed to electronic fields.

It is often suggested that sensitive people do not use wi-fi and connect to the internet by cable. If that does not suit, you could consider switching off your wi-fi at night (although you might still be exposed to that of your neighbours), and using a normal landline handset rather than a cordless phone and a sensible precaution is to not keep your mobile (cell) phone on the body – you could carry it in a bag – and certainly not to sleep with it under your pillow. Many experts advise keeping mobile phones outside the bedroom altogether.

We don't have any proof that EMF has the effect of raising the risk of dementia in humans but you may wish to take precautions anyway.

Hearing loss

Hearing loss is linked to dementia, and older persons with hearing loss are at a higher risk of developing dementia, as was discussed earlier. It is still not completely understood why this is so. It has been postulated (see Chapter 2) that the extra effort of trying to hear when we suffer from hearing loss diverts brain activity away from cognitive effort.

We do know that hearing loss can sometimes be misdiagnosed as dementia. Those with hearing loss may appear to ignore others, have difficulty answering when spoken to and become easily distracted. For this reason if for no other, it is important to address hearing loss and not to ignore it or pretend it is not happening. Many older people like to deny hearing loss as it implies they are 'getting old' or perhaps they may not realise that it is happening. If you constantly have to ask others to repeat themselves or think that those around you are muttering, then consider that the problem may lie with your hearing rather than with others being inconsiderate. There is some current research which is trying to ascertain whether using hearing aids when required mitigates the risk of dementia but until we have the results of this it is worth taking what steps we can to ensure that hearing loss is a risk factor that does not apply to us.

Hearing tests are easy to obtain; most opticians now offer hearing tests as well as eye tests and hearing aids are obtainable in the UK both privately and on the NHS. (If going privately, do make sure not to get devices that are too complicated and sophisticated for the individual to operate. Arthritic hands as well as cognitive issues can make a nonsense of spending a fortune on a cutting-edge device.) It can take a while to get used to hearing aids but those who do this usually assure others that the effort is worth it. If you are serious about avoiding dementia, than pay attention to your hearing and have your hearing tested if others suggest it or if you need to turn up the sound on the radio or TV. If hearing aids are prescribed then be sure to wear them.

Conclusion

In this chapter we have considered some modifiable risk factors – that is, factors which we can act on to minimise them by changing our lifestyle, taking protective action, refusing certain interventions and so on. Some may be easier to tackle than others. Some of these risk factors are better researched than others and some you may dismiss as of no concern to you personally. Once again we need to remember that we are discussing 'risk factors' and to consider how far we are prepared to make changes to reduce our personal risk of developing dementia.

Chapter 11

Modifiable factors: Sleep, stress and social integration

To reduce our risk of developing dementia we can:
- Make changes to increase the quantity and quality of our sleep.
- Look at ways to reduce stress.
- Take three simple steps to start reducing social isolation.

In this chapter we consider three very important factors that may add to or reduce the risk of developing dementia and we consider what we can do to make a difference to each. Quality and quantity of sleep, mitigation of stress and reducing social isolation are all areas of life where any one of us can take direct steps to make a difference.

Sleep

Some research studies have indicated a link between a poor sleep pattern and increased cognitive difficulties.[1] Many older people have trouble sleeping and indeed it is commonly assumed that older people need less sleep for the simple reason that during their waking hours they are not learning new facts or skills and that fewer of their daily experiences involve anything new. (If you follow the recommendations in this book, you *will* be experiencing new things and learning new things, however.)

There are many reasons why sleep patterns may be disturbed in older people: pain from arthritic conditions, discomfort from digestive problems, the need to use the lavatory more frequently and, of course, worry and anxiety commonly experienced by people of any age.

Most of us are aware that a sleepless night has an effect on our functionality the next day but we may not be so aware of the negative effect that long-term poor sleep may have. One such effect is that we miss out on essential 'maintenance' that our brain and body need to perform while we sleep.

Studies suggest that sleep has an essential role in clearing beta-amyloid out of the brain. For example, a small study suggested that losing just one night of sleep led to an increase in beta-amyloid in the brain. Beta-amyloid (or amyloid beta – see page 209) is a metabolic waste product that's found in the fluid between brain cells (neurones and glia, the cells that supply the neurones). A build-up of beta-amyloid is linked to impaired brain function. In Alzheimer's disease, beta-amyloid clumps together to form amyloid plaques, which causes problems with communication between neurones.[2]

Most health advice suggests that the average person needs between seven and nine hours sleep every night. If you habitually get less sleep than this it is worth thinking about increasing your sleep time. However, quality of sleep is also important. A long night of broken sleep can leave you feeling as tired and drained as a curtailed night and it is thought that shallow or broken sleep is not as good for health and wellbeing as several hours of deeper unbroken sleep.

In theory, you know if you are not sleeping well because you feel sleepy during the day, you drop off at odd moments, you feel lethargic and uncoordinated and find it difficult to think straight. However, some people seem to adapt to chronic sleep deprivation and there are always well-known people who claim to need very little sleep and yet can still function day to day. (Margaret Thatcher comes to mind – but she did go on to develop Alzheimer's disease!)

So, assuming that current research findings will be proved to be right as the number of studies increases, and that a lack of sleep is likely to increase our dementia risk, what steps can be taken to ensure that we get the seven to nine hours of sleep recommended? And are there actions that can be taken to improve the quality of the sleep we have?

Ways to improve quantity and quality of sleep

There is some standard advice concerning what is termed 'sleep hygiene'. It is suggested that we should:

- Go to sleep and wake up at regular times, thus educating the body to expect to be sleepy and wakeful by command.
- Keep the bedroom dark.
- Avoid electronic devices in the bedroom. (This includes TVs, tablets, e-readers and mobile phones.) Some experts suggest switching off your internet connection at night.
- Use the bedroom only for sleeping and not for working or other distractions.
- Have a relaxing bedtime routine to 'wind down'.
- Have a cool bedroom.
- Avoid stimulants before bed, such as coffee and alcohol.

This is all good advice as far as it goes, but I think we should look further. The human body is meant to sleep at regular intervals and all new research tends to emphasise the need for this sleep. It is interesting to note that babies and small children

·need (and usually take naturally) more hours of sleep than adults. This seems to indicate that one of the major factors of sleep is the need for the brain to coordinate all the sensations, experiences and connections that have been happening to the individual during the daytime 'waking' hours. Added to this is the new and limited evidence referenced above which suggests that sleep also plays a role in clearing beta-amyloid from the brain. Enabling our brains to do the necessary 'house-keeping' (the technical term is 'autophagy') is clearly very important.

We can address some of the causes of sleeplessness or broken sleep with simple changes.

Electronic devices: It is important to 'wind down' in the hours before retiring to bed and it is especially important to avoid using electronic devices (even checking our phone or email) for at least an hour before we sleep. In this respect, the advice to avoid having electronic devices in the bedroom is sound. There is a caveat here. Many people feel safer keeping the mobile phone nearby in case of emergencies during the night. However, you can avoid charging the phone in your bedroom whilst you are sleeping, keep the phone at a distance from your bed (NEVER sleep with it under your pillow) and switch it into airplane mode or off completely whilst you sleep. In this respect it is probably best to keep bed-time reading to actual books or magazines rather than e-readers.

Avoid bedtime social media and communications: The most important element in getting the prescribed seven to nine hours' sleep is the necessity to calm the mind. In this respect, avoiding looking at phone messages or email is helpful. (Just consider checking your phone to find a worried message from a family member or looking at email and finding a notification of a parking ticket before going to sleep and the effect that is likely to have on your mindset.)

Calming herbal teas: Some people find that a night-time drink of herbal tea is helpful. There are several herbal formulas which are soothing and sleep inducing – chamomile, valerian, hops and lavender for example. Avoid peppermint, and also ginger, as these wake one up, and also any teas that make you more likely to need to go to the lavatory in the night.

Calming the mind: Practising yoga or meditation before bed is helpful but my particular tip is to have as your bedtime reading a soothing book such as a historical diary (think Samuel Pepys or Parson Woodford) or something 'worthy' which you feel you 'ought' to read but which doesn't capture your attention too much. Avoid the latest thriller or anything described as a 'page turner'.

Olfactory stimulation: Some brand new research has found that inhaling pleasant scents using a diffuser during the first two hours of sleep significantly improved cognitive and neural functioning. The researchers found that those inhaling the scents experienced a 226% improvement in memory compared with a control group who received only a trace amount of the diffused scent.[3]

Using light: One tip which I often suggest to my clients who find that their loved one with dementia has trouble settling is to use lights to create a sleep atmosphere. Use lamps (three is a good number) rather than an overhead light. Start the bedtime routine with all lights on and, after performing bedtime ablutions, switch off one lamp as you climb into bed. Switch off the second lamp after settling down and by the time you have finished your bedtime reading (or perhaps listening if you like audiobooks) there is only the last (and dimmest) light to extinguish. The body adapts to reduced light by moving into sleep mode.

Minimise disturbance if you do wake up: Should you wake and feel the need to use the toilet in the night – a major cause of broken sleep in the elderly – there are tips which can help to reduce the disturbance.

- Generally the body adapts to sleep by reducing the action of the kidneys so that we do not need to empty our bladder during the night. When we wake during the night there is a tendency to assume that we need the bathroom but often if you ignore the sensation you will drift back off to sleep without any consequences. You should also resist the temptation to get up to use the bathroom just because your sleeping partner gets up. If going to the toilet is really necessary, it can be helpful to set up small movement-activated night lights which show the way to the bathroom and switch off automatically afterwards. Putting on any light during the night is likely to disturb your sleep pattern so try to avoid this as much as possible. You shouldn't need to consult a clock unless you have medication that needs taking at a set hour (and in this case the best thing is to set an alarm) and the use of movement-activated nightlights should minimise the need to switch on any lamps.

- It used to be suggested that if you found you could not 'drop off' you should get up and go into another room and do something to distract yourself. However, this is not a good idea. By getting up you put your body into 'waking mode' and it will be twice as hard to go back to sleep. Instead, I suggest that you try to enjoy the peace and quiet of the bedroom, keep in mind that you are resting your body even if you are not asleep, and think of something soothing and relaxing such as plans for the garden, recalling a pleasant day out, mulling over the plot of a book, playing a piece of music in your head or quoting a loved piece of poetry. Some people like to pray in the quiet of the night.

If despite all your efforts you find it impossible to get a good seven to nine hours' sleep, then don't make your waking hours worse by worrying about it!

Stress avoidance

We tend to think of stress as a bad thing. People advise us: 'Don't stress about it.' Magazine articles are full of advice about how to avoid stress or how to 'de-stress' ourselves. However, the fact is that up to a point stress is actually good for the mind. Without any stress we would probably never take any action. In the short term, stress and the physical reactions to it help us to cope with a difficult situation. Everyone has heard of the 'fight or flight' response where our brain triggers a physical effect by relaying warnings to the muscles, to tighten them, and to the adrenal glands, to release stress hormones such as adrenaline and cortisol. These hormones help the body prepare to fight or flee to safety: the heart increases its action, blood pressure rises and more blood is sent to the brain and muscles; your breath quickens to get more oxygen into your blood; and your body releases sugars and fats into the blood for energy – to help you fight or run away.

The problem arises when, due to an excess of pressure caused by too many problems or the inability to deal with situations, the body gets 'stuck' in the reaction to stress mode. This can result in physical problems such as an inability to relax or sleep, headaches, digestive problems, heart palpitations, and an increase in minor health difficulties like arthritic pain and back pain. It may also result in cognitive problems, such as an inability to take action (indecisiveness) or to concentrate and a feeling of being 'on edge'.

If you are experiencing the condition often referred to as mild cognitive impairment (MCI), any small problems or difficult situations can be a cause of excess stress. This means that situations which might in the past have simply been minor irritations, such as a faulty household appliance or roadworks that mean you need to find a different route, become major sources of stress. Even those of us not suffering from MCI can get excessively stressed if too many small irritations arise at once or if we are already taken up with a major life event, such as the death of someone close to us.

Of course, one of the major sources of stress is a situation over which we have no control – the Covid pandemic comes to mind. In such a situation, people can get very concerned with small matters – wearing a face covering or avoiding close contact with others – as it gives an illusion of having 'control' over the situation. During the 1939-45 war, for example, many people became heavily involved in volunteering for 'war work' or raising money for 'troop comforts' and it is thought this helped to give them stability in an unstable and out-of-their-control situation.

It is still not clear to scientists whether stress is a cause of dementia or whether the type of person who finds it difficult to cope with stress is more likely to develop dementia anyway. However, from the point of view of avoiding dementia, these differences probably don't matter and what is important is finding a way to cope with excessive stress.

Ways to cope with excessive stress

The two things that cause most stress are the feeling of having too many tasks to complete and the sense of not having control over a situation.

Too much to do

The feeling of having too much to do and the stress caused by it may arise from actually having many things which simultaneously need your attention and input and/or from the feeling that you don't have the time to complete all you need to do. Again, there are simple actions that may make big differences:

- **Make lists and prioritise:** Where there are a large number of tasks looming it can be very helpful to take a few minutes to actually list the things that need doing. Put tasks in order – most important first and least important last. If something really has to be done quickly it should be listed as most important even if it is a minor task. Some people like to go further and allot a 'scale' of importance – most important items numbered higher than least important – but this can over-complicate things. One can then work through the list knowing that the most important or most urgent things are done first and if there is not enough time only the least important are left.

- **Allowing yourself breaks:** As an adjunct to the list it can be worth setting aside a 'task time' of, say, one hour after which you take a short break before continuing through the list – maybe using the break to do something to reward yourself (having a cup of coffee, phoning a friend, reading a chapter of a novel).

- **Break complicated tasks down:** Sometimes it is not the amount that you have to do but the sheer complication of the tasks facing you that causes the stress. In this case it can be helpful to break the task down into a number of steps and just complete one step before taking a break. Often, if you tackle a problem like this, it can suddenly become simple to complete. For example, if there is a problem with the car, you could first simply research on the internet to see if it is likely to be a major fault which needs garage time and money spent or if perhaps it can be 'lived with' for a while until you have more time to deal with the matter.

- **Consider delegating:** If you are good at persuading others you could 'delegate' some tasks but this does mean that you need confidence that the person you have delegated to will really do the job.

Not having control

The biggest cause of stress is the feeling that things are happening over which we have no control. Stress can be reduced by action and the need to take action is one of the first urges that arise in a difficult situation. How often do we find that people give advice such as:

Sue them!

Get compensation!

Write and complain!

It is also true that our friends and family are often very quick to offer help in the form of action:

Let me help?

Can I do that for you?

Do you need a lift/shopping/help with that?

So, taking action (however ineffectual) can reduce stress, but suppose that the situation causing the stress really is beyond your control? Perhaps a partner is ill and in hospital and you have to rely on the healthcare workers to 'take action'. Or perhaps a son or daughter is going through a relationship breakdown and you cannot solve their differences? Or maybe there are financial difficulties caused by outside agencies (the Lloyds crash comes to mind) and you can only await the final outcome?

This kind of stress is the most difficult to deal with as the physical effects of stress – caused by the actions of the brain, the adrenal glands and the hormones coursing through our bodies – are all triggered but they cannot be put to rest by taking action to 'solve the problem'. There are some ways to tackle this:

- **Physical exercise** is one of the first recommendations. This may seem a strange way to solve a mental dilemma but in fact physical exercise can relieve stress, at least in the short term. It can help to relieve your anxiety and clear your mind so that you can think more clearly. You do not have to force yourself into being a 'gym bunny' or taking part in an exercise class if this does not appeal to you. Many people claim that going for a run relieves stress, but even something as simple as taking a walk in pleasant surroundings can be helpful. If the cause of your stress is longer term, then scheduling your exercise session/walk for the same time each day can help to give you something to look forward to. Some people find it helpful to use the walking/running/exercise time to listen to music or perhaps a podcast, but for others the simple act of taking time out to become aware of natural surroundings can be more soothing.

- **Stress-reducing exercise:** There are specific exercise techniques which have a reputation for helping with stress whilst at the same time improving fitness. Yoga, and Tai Chi, are two forms of exercise often recommended, and Qigong, which is becoming better known in western society, claims to make people feel fitter, better balanced, calmer and more able to cope with problems.

- **Diversionary thinking/activity:** Another recommendation is to channel your need for action into something else. Do not be put off by people who may comment that you are 'avoiding the issue' or that you are 'in denial'. Diverting your thoughts and actions into another area is actually a very constructive way of coping with the stress caused by things that are beyond your control. If you are not able to influence the situation that is causing you so much stress, then diverting your thoughts elsewhere is a very positive action. You might, for example, decide to follow a hobby more intensely than before, to take up a new activity, to learn something new or to join a new club. You could combine the benefit of exercise with the benefit of diversion by learning a new exercise technique such as Qigong, as suggested above. The effect of turning your mind away from your current troubles and fixing your thoughts on a completely different subject can help to clarify problems, and diverting thoughts to a new subject refreshes your brain. People often claim that after diverting their thoughts this way their troubles 'fall into place' and cease to be such a major burden. Even if this does not happen to you, your mind will have had a rest from the constant anxiety and everlasting buzzing of worrying thoughts.

- **Mind-calming techniques:** A further suggestion is to make use of meditation techniques such as Mantra meditation or Mindfulness. It may seem counter-productive to take time out to meditate if you feel you are overwhelmed by having too much to do. However, the 'time out' factor can help here as, with a calmer mind, we are more able to prioritise necessary actions and feel capable of attending to what needs doing. Sometimes the very fact of feeling overwhelmed by too many tasks can mean that we do not tackle anything and meditation and especially Mindfulness techniques can make a big difference.

Social integration

Given that we know lack of social integration and avoiding mixing with others are proven risk factors for dementia, we should not be surprised to learn that the 'lockdowns' and social separation forced upon many people by the Covid-19 crisis have led to an increase in the diagnosis of dementia. It will be a few years before we have the facts and figures to corroborate this statement, but those of us working in the field of dementia do not need statistics to convince us. For some people who were in the grey area of 'mild cognitive impairment', the lack of social stimulation may have been critical in leading to a diagnosis of dementia, and those who were in early-stage dementia have inevitably developed worse symptoms.

Carers have been clear in stating to me, 'It all got worse during lockdown' or, 'Once he could not go to his club he became morose and lost interest'.

Mixing with other people, enjoying conversation, taking part in social events and feeling a part of society are all important to lowering the risk of developing dementia. The trouble is that the less we see others and mix with them, the less we may want to do so. It is quite frightening the number of people who have told me that they 'quite enjoyed not having to mix with others' during 2020/21.

It is not necessary to be hugely popular, to have a big circle of friends and acquaintances or, as someone once put it to me to, 'become a party animal' in order to lower the risk factor connected with social integration. People who have a small number of close friends/relatives with whom they feel comfortable and who are willing to share their confidences are just as likely to be considered 'socially integrated' as those who have a huge social circle, are involved in many enterprises and enjoy a varied social life. Interestingly, research has also shown that feeling lonely is not in itself a risk factor for dementia (see page 120). Many people feel lonely at certain periods of their life and the feeling may have no connection with the social life or friendship circle that they move in.

Are there steps we can take to lower this risk factor? It isn't always easy to extend our social circle or to make new friends. Often the friends and acquaintances we make have some connection to us through work or common ground such as our children, our hobbies or simply through frequent contact – how often do you hear people say that they met whilst 'walking the dog'? However, even improving the level of simple social contact – increasing your network of familiar faces such as recognising local people in the street, or the assistant who serves you in the local shop, or knowing who your postman or woman is, or who your neighbours are – can be helpful.

Ways to increase social contact

1. **Be open to 'passing the time of day':** The first step you can take is very easy to initiate. When you are out and about, talk to the people you meet – even if it's only the next-door neighbour or the person on the supermarket checkout. (With the automation of these and the closure of ticket offices, for example, who knows what the consequences for social integration will be!) When you talk to people, they tend to talk back. Often we do not remember to actually have a conversation with others, merely exchanging 'good morning' remarks with a neighbour or simply saying 'thank you' at the checkout when we could ask how they are, for example. As well as being good for our own wellbeing it can lift the spirits of another person if they feel they have been taken notice of and perhaps complimented or even commiserated with.

Covid experience: One client who lived alone told me that when 'lockdown' was imposed she offered to shop for all the people in her cul-de-sac. This she told me was not especially because she wanted to be helpful but because it would ensure that she would talk to some outsider every day when delivering the shopping or accepting the shopping list.

2. **Take active steps to meet others:** Yes, you can stop and chat whilst walking the dog (but we don't all have a dog!), but you could also walk a different route so as to see and greet different dog-walkers. You could choose to shop in different shops – perhaps local shops where you might become known rather than in the big supermarket in town. Go into the local coffee shop – even if you are on your own – and chat to those serving the coffee, those at the next table, those in the queue in front of you. You do not have to initiate a long conversation or interrupt those who are occupied. A simple remark on the weather, 'Goodness, it's cold today', or an opening remark, 'Is it always this busy in here?', will usually get an answer. You are not at this stage looking for a long-term relationship, simply attempting to open yourself up to socialising. Similarly, in community amenities like the public library, you can ask to be directed to books by a certain author or on a certain subject. Assistants in bookshops and garden centres are usually only too pleased to be asked for advice. Their job may be very boring and you will be doing them a favour by introducing some variety into their day.

3. **Take a more active part in events:** Moving on from these beginnings, you might look at any activities, groups or clubs to which you do belong and take a more active part in them. You don't have to become president of the local

Rotary Club (unless you want to, of course), but most clubs and meeting groups will be delighted if you offer to put out chairs, help clear up after meetings, hand out teas and coffees or do the washing up!

What we are discussing here is not a cure for loneliness or a way to make friends – although both of these aims might be what you want. This advice is aimed more at showing how you can extend your part in the social life around you even if you don't want to win the popularity stakes. More social contact will decrease one of the risk factors for developing dementia.

There is a modern tendency to think of our remote (online) social media contacts as 'social integration' but, whilst remote screen contacts can help alleviate loneliness and allow us to keep in contact with those who live some distance away, they do not replace face-to-face contact and conversation. Those who use social media to keep in contact with children and grandchildren will be the first to tell you that it is 'not the same' as meeting up on a family occasion. And for people who actually have dementia, screen contact can be completely meaningless.

In essence then, you can work at increasing your social integration by beginning with these three simple steps. You should find that after the first step it will become much easier to initiate contact with others and the truth is that 'contact leads to more contact' and you will increase your social circle fairly painlessly.

Conclusion

These three factors – sleep, stress and social integration – which are considered to influence our risk of dementia are all areas of life over which we have some control. This means that we can take active steps to lower these risk factors and in doing so we will also be increasing our general wellbeing.

Chapter 12

Thinking ahead

If you are worried that you may have dementia:
- The onset of dementia is not simply 'memory problems'.
- Someone with dementia is unlikely to recognise that they have a problem.
- People who are worried should first see their GP.
- If you have a confirmed diagnosis then now is the time to plan for the future and organise the support you will need.
- Family, neighbours and friends can help, especially if they understand the problems.

What should you do if you think you are developing dementia?

Many, if not most, of us have worries at some time that we are developing cognitive problems. Perhaps it is an increase in those 'senior moments'. Maybe we find that we just cannot grasp how to work a new piece of household equipment. Possibly our family and friends are suggesting that we may have a problem and ought to see a doctor. The popular press is not helpful in the way it describes the first symptoms of dementia. It is common to see statements such as 'dementia begins by forgetting small things such as where we have put our keys'. But forgetting where you have put your keys is not in itself an indication of early dementia. Let us look again at these symptoms:

- Short-term memory loss
- Impaired judgement
- Difficulties with abstract thinking
- Faulty reasoning
- Inappropriate behaviour
- Loss of communication skills
- Disorientation with regard to time and place
- Gait, motor and balance problems
- Neglect of personal care and safety
- Hallucinations, abnormal beliefs, anxiety and agitation.

Unfortunately not everyone in the early stages of dementia is able to understand or realise that they have a problem with cognition. Dementia by its very nature can prevent the clear thinking and analysis of symptoms which might help this realisation. You may think that your memory is fine. Everyone forgets the odd appointment don't they? It is part of getting old. You have not forgotten where you put your wallet. Obviously someone must have moved/stolen it?

If you are not sure whether you have a problem or someone close to you is suggesting that you do, then you might instead like to look at these questions and answer them honestly:

- Does it seem that the person closest to you (wife/ husband/child) is less patient than they used to be?
- Do people accuse you of forgetting appointments (even if you are sure you did not make the appointment)?
- Do you sometimes find that things you use have disappeared from their usual place?
- Do you ever find yourself somewhere without

remembering how you got there?

- Do complete strangers say hello and suggest you were ignoring them?
- Do you feel that you cannot be bothered to do anything?
- Do you lose track of the time quite often?

No one wants to think that they are suffering from a serious disease. Doctors' surgeries are full of patients who did not attend early in their illness because they hoped that by ignoring the symptoms they would go away. For this reason, if your family or friends are saying they are worried about your memory, you should take their concerns seriously. It might help to remember that other conditions can cause memory loss and confusion as discussed in Chapters 1 and X. You may not have dementia. However, if you do have the early stages of dementia it is better to have the diagnosis as soon as possible so that you can get all the support possible.

It may seem that a diagnosis of dementia is a devastating blow, but the time between diagnosis and serious loss of function can also be an opportunity to take stock and remember the important things in life. If you have been diagnosed with dementia or if you are caring for someone who has been, then by all means prepare for the future – but above all, now is the time to enjoy the present. Get the most out of life every day.

References

Introduction

1. Bredesen DE. Reversal of cognitive decline: A novel therapeutic program. *Aging* 2014; 6(9): 707-717. doi: 10.18632/aging.100690
2. Livingston G, Huntley J, Sommerlad A, et al. Dementia prevention, intervention, and care: 2020 report of the Lancet Commission. *Lancet* 2020: 396(10248): 413-446. doi: 10.1016/S0140-6736(20)30367-6.

Chapter 1: Age, personality and social factors

1. NHS. Alzheimer's disease. www.nhs.uk/conditions/alzheimers-disease/ (accessed 4 August 2023)
2. Riley KP, Snowdon DA, Desrosiers MF, Markesbery WR. Early life linguistic ability, late life cognitive function, and neuropathology: Findings from the Nun Study. *Neurobiology of Aging* 2005; 26(3): 341-347. doi:10.1016/j.neurobiolaging.2004.06.019
3. Nicholas H, Moran O, Foy C, et al. Are abnormal premorbid personality traits a marker for Alzheimer's disease? A case-control study. *International Journal of Geriatric Psychiatry* 2010; 25(4): 345-351. doi: 10.1002/gps.2345.
4. McCrae RR, Costa PT. Validation Of the Five-factor Model Of Personality Across Instruments And Observers. *Journal of Personality and Social Psychology* 1987; 1(52): 81-90. doi: 10.1037/0022-3514.52.1.81
5. Field D, Millsap RE. Personality in advanced old age: continuity or change? *J Gerontol* 1991; 46(6): 299-308. doi: 10.1093/geronj/46.6.p299. PMID: 1940085.
6. Kolanowski AM, Whall AL. Life-span perspective of personality in dementia. *Journal of Nursing Scholarship* 1996; 28(4): doi:10.1111/j.1547-5069.1996.tb00380.x

7. Bassuk SS, Glass TA, Berkman LF.Social disengagement and incident cognitive decline in community-dwelling elderly persons. *Annals of Internal Medecine* 1999; 131: 65-173. doi: 10.7326/0003-4819-131-3-199908030-00002

8. Strout KA, Howard E. The Six Dimensions of Wellness and Cognition in Aging Adults. *Journal of Holistic Nursing* 2012; 30(3): 195-204. doi: 10.1177/0898010112440883

9. Lyketsos CG. Cognitive decline in adulthood an 11.5 year follow up of the Baltimore Epidemeological Catchment area study *Am J Psychiatry* 1999; 156: 58-65. doi: 10.1176/ajp.156.1.58

10. Christensen H, Korten AE, Jorm AF, et al. Education and decline in cognitive performance: compensatory but not protective. *Int J Geriatr Psychiatry* 1997; 12(3): 323-330. doi: 10.1002/(SICI)1099-1166(199703)

11. Fairjones SE, Vuletich EJ, Pestell C, Panegyres PK. Exploring the role of cognitive reserve in early onset dementia. *American Journal of Alzheimer's Disease and Other Dementias* 2011; 26(2): 139-144. doi: 10.1177/1533317510397328

12. Stern Y. Cognitive reserve in ageing and Alzheimer's disease. *Lancet Neurol* 2012; doi: 10.1016/S1474-4422(12)70191-6

Chapter 2: Trauma and physical and mental illness

1. Hof PR, Bouras C, Delacourte A, et al. Differential distribution of neurofibrillary tangles in the cerebral cortex of dementia pugilistica and Alzheimer's disease cases. *Acta Neuropathologica* 1992; 85(1): 23-30. doi: 10.1007/BF00304630

2. Plassman BL, Havlik RJ, Steffens DC, et al. Documented head injury in early adulthood and the risk of Alzheimer's disease and other dementias. *Neurology* 2000; 55(8): 1158-1166 doi: 10.1212/wnl.55.8.1158

3. Roberts GW, Gentleman SM, Lynch A, et al. Beta-amyloidprotien deposition in the brain after severe head injury:implications for the pathogenesis of Alzheimer's disease. *J Neurol Neurosurg Psychiatry* 1994; 57(4): 419-425. doi: 10.1136/jnnp.57.4.419

4. Smith DH, Chen X-H, Iwata A, Graham DI. Amyloid-Beta accumulation in axons after traumatic brain injury in humans. *J*

Neurosurg 2003; 98(5): 1072-1077. doi: 10.3171/jns.2003.98.5.1072

5. Nicoll JA, Roberts GW, Graham DI. Apolipoprotein E epsilon4 allele is associated with deposition of amyloid beta-protein following head injury. *Nat Med* 1995; 1(2): 135-137. doi: 10.1038/nm0295-135

6. Mayeux R, Ottman R, Maestre G, et al. Synergistic effects of traumatic head injury and apolipoprotein-epsilon 4 in patients with Alzheimer's disease. *Neurology* 1995; 45(3 Pt 1): 555-557. doi: 10.1212/wnl.45.3.555

7. Lennon MJ, Brooker H, Creese B, et al. Lifetime Traumatic Brain Injury and Cognitive Domain Deficits in Late Life: The PROTECT-TBI Cohort Study. Journal of Neurotrauma . 27 January 2023. doi: 10.1089/neu.2022.0360

8. Carvalho CH, Kimmig H, Lopez WO, et al. Hypertrophic Olivary Degeneration: A Neurosurgical Point of View. *J Neurol Surg A Cent Eur Neurosurg* 2016; 77(1): 59-62. doi/10.1055/s-0035-1566114

9. Blackwell DL, Hayward MD, Crimmins EM. Does childhood health affect chronic morbidity in later life? *Social Science & Medicine* 2001; 52(8): 1269-1284. doi: 10.1016/S0277-9536(00)00230-6

10. Mizrahi EH, Waitzman A, Arad M, Adunsky A. Atrial fibrillation predicts cognitive impairment in patients with ischemic stroke. *Am J Alzheimers Dis Other Demen* 2011; 26(8): 623-626. doi: 10.1177/1533317511432733

11. Diabetes UK. What is diabetes? Getting to know the basics. www.diabetes.org.uk/diabetes-the-basics (accessed 4/9/23)

12. Michailidis M, Moraitou D, Tata DA, Kalinderi K, Papamitsou T, Papaliagkas V. Alzheimer's Disease as Type 3 Diabetes: Common Pathophysiological Mechanisms between Alzheimer's Disease and Type 2 Diabetes. *Int J Mol Sci* 2022; 23(5): 2687. doi: 10.3390/ijms23052687

13. Otto A, Stolk RP, Hofman A, et al. Association of diabetes mellitus and dementia: the Rotterdam Study. *Diabetologia* 1996; 39(11): 1392-1397. doi: 10.1007/s001250050588

14. Pritchard M, Velayudhan L. Cognitive impairment in diabetes patients. *Independent Nurse* 18 February 2014. doi: org/10.12968/indn.2012.16.4.91044

15. Taylor R. Reversing type 2 diabetes and ongoing remission. University of Newcastle. www.ncl.ac.uk/magres/research/

diabetes/reversal/#publicinformation (Accessed 5 October 2023).

16. Itzhaki RF, Lin WR, Shang D, Wilcock GK, Faragher B, Jamieson GA. Herpes simplex virus type 1 in brain and risk of Alzheimer's disease. *Lancet* 1997; 349(9047): 241-244.
doi: 10.1016/S0140-6736(96)10149-5. PMID: 9014911.

17. Murphy MJ, Fani L, Ikram MK, Ghanbari M, Ikram MA. Herpes simplex virus 1 and the risk of dementia: a population-based study. *Sci Rep* 2021; 11(1): 8691. doi: 10.1038/s41598-021-87963-9

18. Klaver CCW, Ott A, Hofman A, et al. Is age-related maculopathy associated with Alzheimer's Disease? The Rotterdam Study. *American Journal of Epidemiology* 1999; 150(9): 963-968.
doi: 10.1093/oxfordjournals.aje.a010105

19. Rong SS, Lee BY, Kuk AK, et al. Comorbidity of dementia and age-related macular degeneration calls for clinical awareness: a meta-analysis. *Br J Ophthalmol* 2019; 103(12): 1777-1783.
doi: 10.1136/bjophthalmol-2018-313277

20. Johnson JCS, Marshall CR, Weil RS, et al. Hearing and dementia: from ears to brains. *Brain* 2021; 144(2): 391-401.
doi: 10.1093/brain/awaa429

21. Ewald PW. *Plague Time: The New Germ Theory of Disease.* Anchor Books, 2002

22. Morales R, Duran-Aniotz C, Castilla J, et al. De novo induction of amyloid beta-deposition. *Molecular Psychiatry* 2012; 17: 1347-1353.
doi: 10.1038/mp.2011.120

23. de Craen AJM, Gussekloo J, Vrijsen B, Westendorp RGJ. Meta-Analysis of Nonsteroidal Antiinflammatory Drug Use and Risk of Dementia. *American Journal of Epidemiology* 2005; 161(2): 114–120.
doi: 10.1093/aje/kwi029

24. Hanning CD. Postoperative cognitive dysfunction. *BJA: British Journal of Anaesthesia* 2005; 95(1): 82–87. doi: 10.1093/bja/aei062

25. Wilson RS, Barnes LL, Mendes de Leon CF, et al. Depressive symptoms, cognitive decline, and risk of AD in older persons. *Neurology* 2002; 59(3): 364-370. doi: 10.1212/wnl.59.3.364

26. Fahim S, van Duijn CM, Baker FM, et al. A study of familial aggregation of depression, dementia and Parkinson's disease. *European Journal of Epidemiology* 1998; 14: 233-238.
doi: 10.1023/a:1007488902983

27. Kessing LV, Andersen PK. Does the risk of developing dementia

increase with the number of episodes in patients with depressive disorder and in patients with bipolar disorder? *J Neurol Neurosurg Psyciatry* 2004; 75(12): 1662-1666. doi: 10.1136/jnnp.2003.031773

28. Gualtieri CT, Johnson LG. Age-related cognitive decline in patients with mood disorders. *Prog Neuropsychopharmacol Biol Psychiatry* 2008; 32(4): 962-967. doi: 10.1016/j.pnpbp.2007.12.030

29. Sokol DK, Maloney B, Long JM, Ray B, Lahiri DK. Autism, Alzheimer disease, and fragile X: APP, FMRP, and mGluR5 are molecular links. *Neurology.* 2011; 76(15):1344-1352. doi: 10.1212/WNL.0b013e3182166dc7

30. Khan SA, Khan SA, Narendra AR, et al. Alzheimer's Disease and Autistic Spectrum Disorder: Is there any Association? *CNS Neurol Disord Drug Targets* 2016; 15(4): 390-402. doi: 10.2174/1871527315666160321104303

31. Pagni BA, Walsh MJM, Ofori E, et al. Effects of age on the hippocampus and verbal memory in adults with autism spectrum disorder: Longitudinal versus cross-sectional findings. *Autism Res* 2022; 15(10): 1810-1823. doi: 10.1002/aur.2797

Chapter 3: Lifestyle choices, miscellaneous factors and risk of dementia

1. Ott A, Slooter AJC, Hofman A, et al. Smoking and risk of dementia and Alzheimer's diseases in a population-based cohort study: the Rotterdam Study. *Lancet* 1998; 351: 1840–1843. doi: 10.1016/s0140-6736(97)07541-7

2. Rusanen M, Kivipelto M, Quesenberry CP, et al. Heavy Smoking in Midlife and Long-term Risk of Alzheimer Disease and Vascular Dementia. *Arch Intern Med* 2011; 171(4): 333-339 doi: 10.1001/archinternmed.2010.393

3. Doll R, Peto R, Boreham J, Sutherland I. Smoking and dementia in male British doctors: prospective study. *Br Med J* 2000; 320(7242): 1097-1102. doi: 10.1136/bmj.320.7242.1097

4. Luchsinger JA, Reitz C, Honig LS, et al. Aggregation of Vascular Risk Factors and Risk of Incident Alzheimer's Disease, *Neurology* 2005; 65(4): 545–551. doi: 10.1212/01.wnl.0000172914.08967.dc

5. Ruitenberg A, van Sweiten JC, Witteman JCM, et al. Alcohol consumption and risk of dementia: the Rotterdam Study. *Lancet*

2002; 359(9303): 281-286. doi: 10.1016/S0140-6736(02)07493-7

6. Letenneur L. Risk of Dementia and Alcohol and Wine Consumption: a review of recent results. *Biol Res* 2004; 37: 189-193. doi: 10.4067/s0716-97602004000200003

7. Lemeshow S, Letenneur L, Dartigues JF, et al. Illustration of analysis taking into account complex survey considerations: the association between wine consumption and dementia in the PAQUID study. *Am J Epidemiol* 1998; 148(3): 298-306. doi: 10.1093/oxfordjournals.aje.a009639

8. Hoang TD, Byers AL, Barnes DE, Yaffe K. Alcohol consumption patterns and coginitive impairment in older women. *Am J Gertiatr Psychiatry* 2014; 22(12): 1663-1667. doi: 10.1016/j.jagp.2014.04.006

9. Laing I, et al. Heavy episodic drinking and risk of cognitive decline in older adults. Presented at Alzheimer's Association International Conference 2012 (AAIC 2012) in Vancouver on Wednesday 18 July. doi: 10.1016/j.jalz.2012.05.1682

10. Sabia S, Fayosse A, Dumurgier J, et al. Alcohol consumption and risk of dementia: 23 year follow-up of Whitehall II cohort study. *Br Med J* 2018; 362: k2927. doi: 10.1136/bmj.k2927

11. Albanese E, Launer LJ, Egger M, et al. Body mass index in midlife and dementia: systematic review and meta-regression analysis of 589,649 men and women followed in longitudinal studies. *Alzheimers Dement (Amst)* 2017; 8: 165–178 doi: 10.1016/j.dadm.2017.05.007

12. Veronese N, Facchini S, Stubbs B, et al. Weight loss is associated with improvements in cognitive function among overweight and obese people: a systematic review and meta-analysis. *Neurosci Biobehav Rev* 2017; 72: 87–94. doi: 10.1016/j.neubiorev.2016.11.017

13. Sabia S, Fayosse A, Dumurgier J, et al. Association of sleep duration in middle and old age with incidence of dementia. *Nat Commun* 2021; 12: 2289. doi: 10.1038/s41467-021-22354-2

14. Shokri-Kojori E, Wang GJ, Wiers CE, et al. β-Amyloid accumulation in the human brain after one night of sleep deprivation. *Proc Natl Acad Sci* 2018; 115(17): 4483-4488. doi: 10.1073/pnas.1721694115

15. Norton MC, Smith KR, Ostbye T, et al., Increased Risk of Dementia When Spouse Has Dementia? TheCache County Study. *J Am Geriatr Soc* 2010 ; 58(5): 895–900. doi: 10.1111/j.1532-5415.2010.02806.x

16. Hao W, Fu C, Zhu D. Early Menopause Is Linked To Increased

Risk Of Presenile Dementia Before Age 65 Years. *Circulation* 2022; 145(S1): AEP67 doi: 10.1161/circ.145.suppl_1.EP67

Chapter 4: Drugs and dementia

1. Elias PK, Elias MF, D'Agostino RB, et al. Serum cholesterol and cognitive performance in the Framingham Heart Study. *Psychosomatic Med* 2005; 67(1): 24-30. doi: 10.1097/01.psy.0000151745.67285.c2.

2. Kennedy RE, Cutter GR, Fowler ME, Schneider LS. Association of concomitant use of cholinesterase inhibitors or memantine with cognitive decline in Alzheimer's clinical trials: a meta-analysis. *JAMA Network Open* 2018; 1(7): e184080.

3. Bredesen D. *The End of Alzheimer's: The first programme to prevent and reverse the cognitive decline of dementia.* Vermilion; 2017.

4. Bredesen DE. Reversal of cognitive decline: A novel therapeutic program. *Aging* 2014; 6(9): 707-717. doi: 10.18632/aging.100690

5. Bredesen DE, Amos EC, Canick J, et al. Reversal of cognitive decline in Alzheimer's disease. *Aging* 2016: 8(6): 1250-1258

6. Bredesen DE, Sharlin K, Jenkins D, et al. Reversal of cognitive decline: 100 patients. *J of Alzheimer's Disease and Parkinsonism* 2018; 85(5): 450.

7. Haynes A. 36 'Holes in the Roof': The Dawn of the Era of Treatable and Preventable Alzheimer's Disease. *Clinical Education* 25 March 2015. www.clinicaleducation.org/resources/reviews/36-holes-in-the-roof-the-dawn-of-the-era-of-treatable-and-preventable-alzheimers-disease/

8. Graveline D. *Lipitor: Thief of Memory* Duane Graveline, 2006

9. Gaist D. Statins and the risk of polyneuropathy: A Case-Control study. *Neurology* 2002; 58(9): 1333-1337.

10. Golomb BA, Verden A, Messner AK, et al. Amyotrophic Lateral Sclerosis associated with Statin Use: A Disproportionality Analysis of the FDA's Adverse Event Reporting System. *Drug Safety* 2018; 41: 403-413.

11. Padala KP, Padala PR, McNeilly, et al. The effect of HMG-CoA reductase inhibitors on cognition in patients with Alzheimer's dementia: a prospective withdrawal and rechallenge pilot study. *American Journal of Geriatric Pharmacotherapy* 2012; 10(5): 296-302.

doi: 10.1016/j.amjopharm.2012.08.002

12. McGuiness B, Craig D, Bullock R, Passmore P. Statins for the prevention of dementia. *Cochrane Database of Systematic Reviews* 2016; 1: Art. CD003160 doi: 10.1002/14651858.CD003160.pub3

13. Xie Y, Bowe B, Li T, et al. Risk of death among users of proton pump inhibitors: a longitudinal observational study of United States veterans. BMJ Open 2017; 7(6): e015735. doi: 10.1136/bmjopen-2016-015735

14. Zhang Y, Liang M, Sun C, et al. Proton pump inhibitors use and dementia risk: a meta-analysis of cohort studies. *Eur J Clin Phramcol* 2020; 76(2): 139-147. doi: 10.1007/s00228-019-02753-7

15. Gomm W, von Holt K, Thome F, et al. Association of proton pump inhibitors with risk of dementia: A pharmacoepidemiological claims data analysis. *JAMA Network* 2016; 73(4): 410-416. doi: 10.1001/jamaneurol.2015.4791

16. Richardson K, Fox C, Maidment I, et al. Anticholinergic drugs and risk of dementia: case-control study. *Br Med J* 2018; 361: k1315. doi: 10.1136/bmj.k1315

17. Gray SL, Anderson ML, Dublin A, et al. Cumulative use of strong anticholinergics and incident dementia: a prospective cohort study. *JAMA Int Med* 2015; 175: 401-407. doi: 10.1001/jamainternmed.2014.7663

18. Pase MP, Himali JJ, Beiser AS, et al. Sugar- and artificially sweetened beverages and the risks of incident stroke and dementia. *Stroke* 2017; 48: 1139-1141. doi: 10.1161/STROKEAHA.116.016027

Chapter 5: Nutrition and dodging dementia

1. FAO, IFAD, UNICEF, WFP and WHO. 2020. In Brief to The State of Food Security and Nutrition in the World 2020. Transforming food systems for affordable healthy diets. Rome, FAO. doi: 10.4060/ca9699en

2. Pasinetti GM, Eberstein JA. Metabolic syndrome and the role of dietary lifestyles in Alzheimer's disease. *J Neurochem* 2008; 106: 1503-1514. doi: 10.1111/j.1471-4159.2008.05454.x

3. Seneff S, Wainwright G, Mascitelli L.. Nutrition and Alzheimer's disease: The detrimental role of a high carbohydrate diet. *Eur J Intern Med* 2011; 22(2): 134-140. doi:10.1016/j.ejim.2010.12.017

4. Quin W, Chachich M, Lane M, et al.Calorie restriction attenuates Alzheimer's disease type brain amyloidosis in Squirrel monkeys (Saimiri sciureus). *J Alzheimers Dis* 2006; 10(4): 417-422. doi: 10.3233/jad-2006-10411

5. Barnes LL, Dhana K, Liu X, et al. Trial of the MIND Diet for Prevention of Cognitive Decline in Older Persons. *New England Journal of Medicine* 2023; 389: 602-611. doi: 10.1056/NEJMoa2302368

6. de Rooij SR, Wouters H, Yonker JE, Roseboom TJ. Prenatal undernutrition and cognitive function in late adulthood. *PNAS* 2010; 107(39): 16881-16886. doi: 10.1073/pnas.1009459107

7. Djuricic I, Calder PC. Beneficial Outcomes of Omega-6 and Omega-3 Polyunsaturated Fatty Acids on Human Health: An Update for 2021. *Nutrients* 2021; 13(7): 2421. doi: 10.3390/nu13072421. PMID: 34371930; PMCID: PMC8308533.

8. Dangour AD, Allen E, Elbourne D, Fletcher A, Richards M, Uauy R. Fish consumption and cognitive function among older people in the UK: baseline data from the OPAL study. *J Nutr Health Aging* 2009; 13(3): 198-202. doi: 10.1007/s12603-009-0057-2. PMID: 19262951.

9. Newton M. *Alzheimer's: What if there was a cure?* Basic Health Publications; 2013.

9a. de la Rubia Ortí JE, García-Pardo MP, Drehmer E,et al. Improvement of Main Cognitive Functions in Patients with Alzheimer's Disease after Treatment with Coconut Oil Enriched Mediterranean Diet: A Pilot Study. *J Alzheimers Dis* 2018; 65(2): 577-587. doi: 10.3233/JAD-180184. PMID: 30056419.

10. Van der Auwera I, Wera S, Van Leuven F, Henderson ST. A ketogenic diet reduces amyloid beta 40 and 42 in a mouse model of Alzheimer's disease. *Nutr Metab (Lond)* 2005; 2: 28. doi: 10.1186/1743-7075-2-28. PMID: 16229744

11. Henderson ST, Vogel JL, Barr LJ, Garvin F, Jones JJ, Costantini LC. Study of the ketogenic agent AC-1202 in mild to moderate Alzheimer's disease: a randomized, double-blind, placebo-controlled, multicenter trial. *Nutr Metab (Lond)* 2009; 6: 31. doi: 10.1186/1743-7075-6-31. PMID: 19664276.

12. McCleery J, Abraham RP, Denton DA, Rutjes AWS, Chong L, Al-Assaf AS, Griffith DJ, Rafeeq S, Yaman H, Malik MA, Di Nisio

M, Martínez G, Vernooij RWM, Tabet N. Vitamin and mineral supplementation for preventing dementia or delaying cognitive decline in people with mild cognitive impairment. *Cochrane Database of Systematic Reviews* 2018; 11. Art. No. CD011905. doi: 10.1002/14651858.CD011905.pub2

13. Rutjes AW, Denton DA, Di Nisio M, Chong LY, Abraham RP, Al-Assaf AS, Anderson JL, Malik MA, Vernooij RW, Martínez G, Tabet N, McCleery J. Vitamin and mineral supplementation for maintaining cognitive function in cognitively healthy people in mid and late life. *Cochrane Database Syst Rev* 2018; 12(12): CD011906. doi: 10.1002/14651858.CD011906.pub2. PMID: 30556597.

14. Martínez GV, Salas AA, Ballestín SS. Vitamin Supplementation and Dementia: A Systematic Review. *Nutrients* 2022; 14(5): 1033. doi: 10.3390/nu14051033. PMID: 35268010; PMCID: PMC8912288.

15. Lu'o'ng KV, Nguyên LT. The beneficial role of vitamin D in Alzheimer's disease. *Am J Alzheimers Dis Other Demen* 2011; 26(7): 511-520. doi: 10.1177/1533317511429321. PMID: 22202127.

16. Sano M, Ernesto C, Thomas RG, et al. A controlled trial of selegiline, alpha-tocopherol, or both as treatment for Alzheimer's disease. The Alzheimer's Disease Cooperative Study. *N Engl J Med* 1997; 336(17): 1216-1222. doi: 10.1056/NEJM199704243361704.

17. Le Bars PL, Velasco FM, Ferguson JM, et.al. Influence of the Severity of Cognitive Impairment on the Effect of the Ginkgo biloba Extract EGb 761 in Alzheimer's Disease. *Neuropsychobiology* 2002; 45(1): 19–26. doi: 10.1159/000048668

18. DeKosky ST, Williamson JD, Fitzpatrick AL, et al. Ginkgo Evaluation of Memory (GEM) Study Investigators. Ginkgo biloba for prevention of dementia: a randomized controlled trial. *JAMA* 2008; 300(19): 2253-2262. doi: 10.1001/jama.2008.683. Erratum in: *JAMA* 2008; 300(23): 2730. PMID: 19017911; PMCID: PMC2823569.

19. Brondino N, De Silvestri A, Re S, Lanati N, et al. A Systematic Review and Meta-Analysis of Ginkgo biloba in Neuropsychiatric Disorders: From Ancient Tradition to Modern-Day Medicine. *Evid Based Complement Alternat Med* 2013; 2013: 915691. doi: 10.1155/2013/915691. PMID: 23781271; PMCID: PMC3679686.

20. Weinreb O, Mandel S, Amit T, Youdim MBH. Neurological mechanisms of green tea polyphenols in Alzheimer's and Parkinson's diseases. *Journal of Nutritional Biochemistry* 2004; 15(9):

506-516. doi: 10.1016/j.jnutbio.2004.05.002

21. Feng L, Cheah IK, Ng MM, Li J, Chan SM, Lim SL, Mahendran R, Kua EH, Halliwell B. The Association between Mushroom Consumption and Mild Cognitive Impairment: A Community-Based Cross-Sectional Study in Singapore. *J Alzheimers Dis* 2019; 68(1): 197-203. doi: 10.3233/JAD-180959. PMID: 30775990.

Chapter 6: Assessing personal risk – Genetics and your personal history of trauma, mental health problems and physical disease

1. Thomson J. *Curing The Incurable – Beyond the Limits of Medicine.* London, UK: Hammersmith Health Books; 2020.

2. Van Der Kolk B. *The Body Keeps the Score.* London, UK: Penguin Books; 2014.

3. Easthope L. *When The Dust Settles.* London, UK: Hodder and Stoughton; 2022.

4. Persson S. *Smallpox, Syphilis and Salvation: Medical Breakthroughs That Changed the World.* ReadHowYouWant.com; 2010.p.

5. Broxmeyer L. *Alzheimer's Disease — How Its Bacterial Cause Was Found and Then Discarded.* CreateSpace, 2016

6. Ostlund G, Borg K, Wahlin A. Cognitive functioning in post-polio patients with and without general fatigue. *J Rehabil Med* 2005; 37(3): 147-151. doi: 10.1080/16501970410024172. PMID: 16040471.

7. Ott A, Stolk RP, Hofman A, van Harskamp F, Grobbee DE, Breteler MM. Association of diabetes mellitus and dementia: the Rotterdam Study. *Diabetologia* 1996; 39(11): 1392-1397. doi: 10.1007/s001250050588. PMID: 8933010

8. Pritchard M, Velayudhan L. Cognitive impairment in diabetes patients. *Independent Nurse* 2014; 2012(4): doi: 10.12968/indn.2012.16.4.91044

9. Americal Academy of Neuorlogy. Thyroid problems linked to increased risk of dementia. *Science Daily* 6 July 2022. www.sciencedaily.com/releases/2022/07/220706165418.htm

10. Elbadawy AM, Mansour AE, Abdelrassoul IA, Abdelmoneim RO. Relationship between thyroid dysfunction and dementia. *The Egyptian Journal of Internal Medicine* 2020; 32: 9.

doi: 10.1186/s43162-020-00003-2

11. Gendelman O, Tiosano S, Shoenfeld Y, et al. High proportions of dementia among SLE patients: A big data analysis. *Geriatric Psychiatry* 2017; 33(3): 531-536. doi: 10.1002/gps.4819

12. Park H, Yim DH, Ochirpurev B, et al. Association between dementia and systemic rheumatic disease: A nationwide population-based study. *PLoS One* 2021; 16(3): e0248395. doi: 10.1371/journal.pone.0248395

13. Sangha PS, Thakur M, Akhtar Z, et al. The Link Between Rheumatoid Arthritis and Dementia: A Review. *Cureus* 2020; 12(4): e7855. doi:10.7759/cureus.7855

14. Rong SS, Lee BY, Kuk AK, et al. Comorbidity of dementia and age-related macular degeneration calls for clinical awareness: a meta-analysis. *British Journal of Ophthalmology* 2019; 103: 1777-1717. doi: 10.1136/bjophthalmol-2018-313277

Chapter 7: Assessing your current status

1. Livingston G, Huntley J, Sommerlad A. Dementia prevention, intervention, and care: 2020 report of the Lancet Commission. *Lancet* 2020; 396(10248): 413-446. doi: 10.1016/S0140-6736(20)30367-6

2. Albanese E, Launer LJ, Egger M, et al. Body mass index in midlife and dementia: systematic review and meta-regression analysis of 589,649 men and women followed in longitudinal studies. *Alzheimer's Dement (Amst)* 2017; 8: 165–178.

3. Sommerlad A, Ruegger J, Singh-Manoux A, Lewis G, Livingston G. Marriage and risk of dementia: systematic review and meta-analysis of observational studies. *J Neurol Neurosurg Psychiatry* 2018; 89: 231–238.

4. Penninkilampi R, Casey AN, Singh MF, Brodaty H. The association between social engagement, loneliness, and risk of dementia: a systematic review and meta-analysis. *J Alzheimers Dis* 2018; 66: 1619–1633.

5. Bell G, Singham T, Saunders R, John A, Stott J. Positive psychological constructs and association with reduced risk of mild cognitive impairment and dementia in older adults: A systematic review and meta-analysis. *Ageing Research Reviews* 2022; 77:101594. doi: 10.1016/j.arr.2022.101594

Chapter 8: Nutrition – What should I eat?

1. Lorin H. *Alzheimer's Solved*. BookSurge Publishing; 2006.
2. Buxton J. *The Great Plant-Based Con*. Piatkus; 2022.
3. Vogiatzoglou A, Refsum H, Johnston C, Smith SM, et al. Vitamin B12 status and rate of brain volume loss in community-dwelling elderly. Neurology 2008; 71(11): 826-832. doi: 10.1212/01.wnl.0000325581.26991.f2
4. Lechinsky H, Afshini A, Ashbaugh C, et al. Health effects associated with consumption of unprocessed red meat: a Burden of Proof study. *Nat Med* 2022; 28: 2075-2082.
5. Mohajeri MH, Troesch B, Weber P. Inadequate supply of vitamins and DHA in the elderly: implications for brain aging and Alzheimer-type dementia. *Nutrition* 2015; 31(2): 261-275. doi: 10.1016/j.nut.2014.06.016
6. Nguyen PK, Lin S, Heidenreich P. A systematic comparison of sugar content in low-fat vs regular versions of food. *Nutr Diabetes* 2016; 6(1): e193. doi: 10.1038/nutd.2015.43
7. Van Tulleken C. *Ultra Processed People: Why Do We All Eat Stuff That Isn't Food…and Why can't We Stop*. Cornerstone Press: 2023.

Chapter 9: Exercise for body and brain

1. NHS Choices. Benefits of exercise. NHS 2022. (Accessed March 2022 - web page no longer available)
2. Colcombe SJ, Erickson KI, Scalf PE, et al. Aerobic exercise training increases brain volume in aging humans. *Journals of Gerontology: Series A – Biological Sciences and Medical Sciences* 2006; 61(11): 1166-1170. doi: 10.1093/gerona/61.11.1166.
3. Laurin D, Verreault R, Lindsay J, et Al. Physical activity and the risk of cognitive impairment and dementia in elderly persons. *Archives of Neurology* 2001; 58(3): 498-504. doi: 10.1001/archneur.58.3.498
4. Cotman C W, Berchtold NC. Exercise: a behavioural intervention to enhance brain health and plasticity. *Trends in Neuroscience* 2002; 25: 295-301. doi: 10.1016/s0166-2236(02)02143-4
5. Jedrziewski MK, Ewbank DC, Wang H, Trojanowski, JQ. Exercise and cognition: results from the National Long Term Care Survey. *Alzheimer's and Dementia* 2010; 6(6): 448-455.

doi: 10.1016/j.jalz.2010.02.004

6. Andel R, Crowe M, Pedersen NL, et al. Physical exercise at midlife and risk of dementia three decades later: a population-based study of Swedish twins. *J Gerontol Series A: Biol Sci Med Sci* 2008; 63(1): 62-66. doi: 10.1093/gerona/63.1.62

7. Snowdon D. *Aging with Grace: The Nun Study and the science of old age*. Fourth Estate; 2011.

8. Honea RA, Thomas GP, Harsha A, et al. Cardiorespiratory fitness and preserved medial temporal lobe volume in Alzheimer disease. *Alzheimer Disease and Associated Disorders* 2009; 23: 188-197. doi: 10.1097/WAD.0b013e31819cb8a2

9. Lautenschlager NT, Cox KL, Flicker L, et al. Effect of physical activity on cognitive function in older adults at risk of Alzheimer disease: a randomized trial. *Journal of the American Medical Association* 2008; 300: 1027-1037. doi: 10.1001/jama.300.9.1027

10. Scarmeas N, Luchsinger JA, Schupf N, et al. Physical activity, diet and risk of Alzheimer disease. *Journal of the American Medical Association* 2009; 302(6): 627-637. doi: 10.1001/jama.2009.1144

11. Heyn P, Abreu BC, Ottenbacher KJ. The effects of exercise training on elderly persons with cognitive impairment and dementia: a meta-analysis. *Archives of Physical Medicine and Rehabilitation* 2004; 85: 1694-1704. doi: 10.1016/j.apmr.2004.03.019

12. Baker LD. Effects of aerobic exercise on mild cognitive impairment: A controlled trial. *Archives of Neurology* 2010; 67(1): 71-79. doi: 10.1001/archneurol.2009.307

13. Teri L, Gibbons LE, McCurry SM, et al. Exercise plus behavioural management in patients with Alzheimer's disease: A randomized controlled trial. *Journal of the American Medical Association* 2003; 290: 2015-2022. doi: 10.1001/jama.290.15.2015

13a. Sturman MT, Morris MC, Mendes de Leon CF, Bienias JL, Wilson RS, Evans DA. Physical activity, cognitive activity, and cognitive decline in a biracial community population. *Arch Neurol* 2005; 62(11): 1750-1754.
doi: 10.1001/archneur.62.11.1750. PMID: 16286550.

14. Stern Y. Cognitive reserve in ageing and Alzheimer's disease. *Lancet Neurol* 2012; 11(11): 1006–1012.
doi: 10.1016/S1474-4422(12)70191-6

15. Leanos S, Kürüm E, Strickland-Hughes CM, et al. The Impact of

Learning Multiple Real-World Skills on Cognitive Abilities and Functional Independence in Healthy Older Adults. *The Journals of Gerontology: Series B* 2020; 75(6): 1155–1169.
doi: 10.1093/geronb/gbz084

16. Walking Football. Walking Football Association England. https://thewfa.co.uk (accessed 21 July 2023)

Chapter 10: Modifiable risk factors – Alcohol, air pollution, smoking, vaping, infections, falls, hospital admissions, elective surgery, EMFs and hearing loss

1. Ruitenberg A, van Swieten JC, Wittman JSM, et al. Alcohol consumption and risk of dementia:the Rotterdam study, *Lancet* 2002; 359: doi: 10.1016/S0140-6736(02)07493-7

2. Sabia S, Fayosse A, Dumurgier J, et al. Alcohol consumption and risk of dementia: 23 year follow-up of Whitehall II cohort study. *BMJ* 2018; 362: k2927. doi: 10.1136/bmj.k2927

3. Oudin A, Segersson D, Adolfsson R, Forsberg B. Association between air pollution from residential wood burning and dementia incidence in a longitudinal study in Northern Sweden. *PLoS One* 2018; 13(6): e0198283. doi: 10.1371/journal.pone.0198283

4. Oudin A, Forsberg B, Adolfsson AN, et al. Traffic-related air pollution and dementia incidence in northern Sweden: a longitudinal study. *Environ Health Perspect* 2016; 124(3): 306–312. doi: 10.1289/ehp.1408322

5. Carey IM, Anderson HR, Atkinson RW, et al. Are noise and air pollution related to the incidence of dementia? A cohort study in London, England. *BMJ Open* 2018; 8(9): e022404. doi: 10.1136/bmjopen-2018-022404

6. Darville A, Hahn EJ. E-cigarettes and Atherosclerotic Cardiovascular Disease: What Clinicians and Researchers Need to Know. *Curr Atheroscler Rep* 2019; 21: 15. doi: 10.1007/s11883-019-0777-7

7. Creditor MC. Hospitalisation leading to 'irreversible functional decline – Hazards of hospitalization of the elderly. *Annals of Internal Medicine* 1993; 118(3): 219-223.

doi: 10.7326/0003-4819-118-3-199302010-00011

8. Møllgård K, Beinlich FRM, Kusk P, et al. A mesothelium divides the subarachnoid space into functional compartments. *Science* 2023; 379(6627): 84-88. doi: 10.1126/science.adc8810. PMID: 36603070.

9. Beason RC, Semm P. Responses of neurons to an amplitude modulated microwave stimulus. *Neurosci Lett* 2002; 333(3): 175-178. doi: 10.1016/s0304-3940(02)00903-5

10. Miller AB, Sears ME, Morgan LL, et al. Risks to Health and Well-Being From Radio-Frequency Radiation Emitted by Cell Phones and Other Wireless Devices. *Front Public Health* 2019; 7: 223. doi: 10.3389/fpubh.2019.00223

11. Goldsworth A. The Biological Effects of Weak Electromagnetic Fields: Problems and solutions. March 2012. https://ehtrust.org/wp-content/uploads/Goldsworthy-2012.pdf (accessed 21 July 2023)

Chapter 11: Modifiable factors – Sleep, stress and social integration

1. Yaffe K, Laffan AM, Harrison SL, et al. Sleep-disordered breathing, hypoxia, and risk of mild cognitive impairment and dementia in older women. *Journal of the American Medical Association* 2011; 306(6): 613-619. doi: 10.1001/jama.2011.1115

2. Shokri-Kojori E, Wang G-J, Wiers CE, et al. β-Amyloid accumulation in the human brain after one night of sleep deprivation. Proc Natl Acad Sci USA 2018; 115(17): 4483-4488. doi: 10.1073/pnas.1721694115

3. Woo CC, Miranda B, Sathishkumar M, Dehkordi-Vakil F, Yassa MA, Leon M. Overnight olfactory enrichment using an odorant diffuser improves memory and modifies the uncinate fasciculus in older adults. *Front Neurosci* 2023; 17: 1200448. doi: 10.3389/fnins.2023.1200448

Glossary

Alzheimer's disease: The most common cause of dementia, characterised by *gradual* decline in mental processes, generally starting with disorientation, short-term memory loss and loss of motivation. The brain characteristically shows plaques of the protein **amyloid beta** and **neurofibrillary tangles**.

Amyloid beta (aka beta-amyloid): A protein (peptide) that is essential to normal brain functioning but which is thought to cause Alzheimer's disease by building up into insoluble 'plaques' in the brain.

Amyloidosis: A condition where amyloid proteins are abnormally deposited in organs or tissues and cause harm.

Amino acids: Organic chemicals which mix in various combinations to make protein.

Astrocytes: Characteristic star-shaped cells found in the brain and spinal cord.

Atrial fibrillation: An erratic (fast and irregular) heartbeat.

Axon: A long slender projection from a nerve cell which carries electrical impulses away from the nerve body.

Case-control study: Research where each participant receiving the active intervention (or attribute) being studied is matched by a 'control' participant who is similar in all respects other than the intervention or attribute being studied.

Chromosome: An organised structure of DNA and protein found in the nucleus of each living cell. Humans have 23 pairs of chromosomes, each of which consists of genetic coding and other regulatory material that together encodes the development of the individual.

Cognition: The mental processes, including attention, memory, language production and understanding, problem solving, planning and decision making.

Cognitive reserve: The resistance of the mental processes to damage from trauma and/or disease.

Dementia: An umbrella term for the group of symptoms that characterise more than 60 different conditions, of which Alzheimer's disease is the most common.

Dementia with Lewy bodies: Dementia where the brain shows tiny spherical deposits (Lewy bodies) that develop in nerve cells, interrupting the action of chemical messengers.

Dendrites: Thread-like extensions of brain cells (neurons) that connect to other neurons and develop with learning.

Fronto-temporal dementia: An umbrella term for dementias arising from damage to the frontal lobes of the brain, including Pick's disease, frontal or temporal lobe degeneration, and dementia associated with motor neurone disease.

Gene: A single element in the coding found in each cell in the body that dictates how that cell, and hence the whole person, should develop.

Hippocampus: A part of the cortex of the human brain that is responsible for consolidating short-term memory as long-term memory, and for spatial organisation. It is one of the first parts of the brain to be affected in Alzheimer's disease. Its name relates to its shape; 'hippos' is the Ancient Greek for 'horse', and 'campus' for 'sea monster' – in other words, 'sea horse'.

Infarct: Death of body tissue due to shutting off the blood supply, as for example in a stroke.

Ischaemia: A decrease in the blood supply to a bodily organ, tissue, or part caused by constriction or obstruction of the blood vessels by a blood clot.

Ketones: One of a group of organic compounds produced during the metabolism of fats.

Lewy body dementia – see **Dementia with Lewy bodies**.

Mild cognitive impairment (MCI): Cognitive impairment, especially short-term memory loss, beyond what would be expected given age and education, but which is not significant enough to interfere with the activities of everyday living.

Mini-Mental State Examination (MMSE): A 30-item questionnaire that is used to screen for impairment to mental processes and to assess decline in mental processes over time. It also called the 'Folstein test'.

Myelin: The fatty substance that forms a covering 'sheath' around the **axons** of nerve cells and facilitates the passage of electrical impulses through those cells.

Neural reserve: Spare capacity in the brain, in the shape of nerve cells, multiple linkages between nerve cells, and networks, that allows the brain to compensate for the effects of disease, trauma and aging.

Neurofibrillary tangles: Aggregations of a protein called 'tau' that are the primary markers, along with **amyloidosis**, in the brain of Alzheimer's disease.

Neuron: Nerve cells that make up the brain, spinal cord and peripheral nervous system. They consist of a cell body, containing the cell nucleus, a long tail (the **axon**) and many branching connections (**dendrites**) to other neurons.

Neuroplasticity: The brain's ability to reorganise itself by forming new neural connections throughout life.

Neurotransmitters: Chemical substances released from nerve endings to transmit impulses to other nerve cells (**neurons**). They include adrenaline (now generally called 'epinephrine'), dopamine and serotonin.

Non-steroidal anti-inflammatory drugs (NSAIDs): A class of drugs, such as aspirin and ibuprofen, that provide pain relief, reduce fever and, at high doses, reduce inflammation, but are not steroids.

Pathogenesis: The process that leads to the development of a disease.

Plaques - See **Amyloid beta**.

Prion diseases: Rare, fatal neurodegenerative disorders caused by misfolded prion proteins (PrP) in the brain.

Prostaglandins: Hormone-like substances present in tissues and body fluids that act as important chemical messengers or mediators. Unlike hormones, which are produced by specialised organs in the body, prostaglandins are produced, and act, locally.

Randomised controlled trial: This describes research that is carried out in a way that is regarded as the gold standard in clinical science, especially for assessing the efficacy of new treatments. 'Randomised' refers to the fact that participants in the trial ('subjects') are randomly allocated to either the treatment group or the 'control' group; they are not deliberately chosen for one or the other. 'Controlled' refers to there being equal numbers of active subjects (who receive the new drug, for example) and 'controls' who receive an imitation of the drug (a 'placebo'). If a trial is also described as 'blinded', or 'double-blinded', this means that neither the participants nor the researchers know who has been allocated to receive the active intervention or the placebo.

Spirochaetes: Spiral shaped bacteria that lack a rigid cell wall and move by means of muscular flexion.

Statins: Medicines that can help lower the level of low-density lipoprotein (LDL) cholesterol in the blood.

Synapse: The minute gap between the nerve endings of one **neuron** and those of another, across which neurons communicate by passing **neurotransmitters** from one to another.

Transient ischaemic attacks (TIAs): Sometimes called 'mini strokes', these are episodes when insufficient blood reaches the brain for such a short time it is barely noticeable, though the effects may be similar to those of a full scale stroke.

Vascular dementia: Dementia that arises from problems with the supply of blood to the brain, typically from a series of **infarcts**. It is characterised by a stepped decline in mental processes, and is the second most common form of dementia.

Sources of help, advice and support in the UK

Adapt Dementia Ltd
Founded by Mary Jordan and a fellow health professionals
with years of direct experience working in dementia care and
support between us. We especially want to allow families living
with dementia to be better informed and to have a wide choice
of support. We believe strongly that everyone has the right
to choose for themselves the therapies, support options and
lifestyle that suits their own experience of dementia. For us
there is no 'one size fits all' solution.
https://www.adaptdementia.com/contact-us/

Alzheimer's Society
A registered charity operating within England and Wales that
provides information and raises money for research into all
types of dementia. There is also a 'hands on' support service
which helps people who have a dementia diagnosis. Different
levels of service are provided in different areas depending upon
funding. Normally services are not offered to people without
an 'official' diagnosis of some form of dementia but information
on the website is accessible to anyone. There are links to other
services.
https://www.alzheimers.org.uk

Alzheimer's Scotland
Working to ensure no one in Scotland faces dementia alonge.
https://www.alzscot.org

Citizens' Advice
A network of independent charities offering confidential advice online, over the phone, and in person, free. They claim to be independent and totally impartial. You can check their website or visit one of their local centres in person or obtain telephone advice on a range of problems. One big beneficial aspect is that if they do not actually deal with the problem you have they will direct you to a service which can help you
www.Citizensadvice.org.uk

Independent Living
Website providing impartial information about living independently with a disability. They are not part of a charity or government organisation. The site provides information on products and services and users can sign up to a weekly email news roundup. This site does not deal exclusively with memory problems or dementia-related issues but there is plenty of information about these areas. They do have a dedicated website area for cognitive issues:
https://www.independentliving.co.uk/il-editorials/dementia-cognitive-impairment/

Walking Football and Walking Netball
Games played at walking pace, with players not allowed to run. It gives an opportunity for older people to stay fit enjoying the games of their youth.
https://thewfa.co.uk/
https://www.englandnetball.co.uk/

Specific problems

Hearing loss
A site that lets you test your hearing and practice to improve.
www.eargym.world

Help with technology
Free technological support and information – includes home visits
www.abilitynet.org.uk

Stroke
Advice and information on recovery from stroke
www.stroke.org.uk

Acknowledgements

This has been a difficult book to write mainly because, even as we went to press, new research papers were coming to the public eye. It will be clear to the reader that some of my conclusions have been based on personal experience (this has been clearly stated in the text where appropriate) but all the while the specific evidence continues to be nebulous, I need make no apology for this.

I am so glad to have worked with Jerry Thompson who has given us such a clear viewpoint on the part that drugs may play in causing symptoms and who has answered all my queries with courtesy and kindness.

I need to thank Carrie Wright and Tristram Jordan for some help with tidying the text and references before publication and give a massive thanks to Georgina Bentliff of Hammersmith Health Books who has encouraged and corrected me, borne with my tardiness and been a kind mentor on occasion.

I owe most thanks of course to my many clients and contacts – both those with dementia and those caring for them – who have given me such insight into the lifestyles and experiences which may have a bearing on the lead up to diagnosis.

Index

Note: AD is the abbreviation for Alzheimer's disease. Glossary page numbers are in bold.

Note: AD is the abbreviation for Alzheimer's disease. Glossary page numbers are in bold.

Note: AD is the abbreviation for Alzheimer's disease. Glossary page numbers are in bold.

Note: AD is the abbreviation for Alzheimer's disease. Glossary page numbers are in bold.

Index

Note: AD is the abbreviation for Alzheimer's disease. Glossary page numbers are in bold.

Note: AD is the abbreviation for Alzheimer's disease. Glossary page numbers
are in bold.

postoperative delirium, 36, 168
symptoms and signs of early-stage dementia, 190
synapses, 68, **213**
  and brain plasticity, 15
systemic inflammation, 36
systemic lupus erythematosus (SLE), 104–105

tacrine, 59
tai chi, 116, 183
tasks, too many, 180–182
teas
  green, 88
  herbal, 177
temporal lobes, 14, 106, 150
thiamine deficiency and alcohol, 47–48
thinking *see* thoughts and thinking
This is Me document (Alzheimer's Society UK), 166
thoughts and thinking
  diversionary, 183–184
  thought processes, 16
thyroid problems, 103–104
TNF (tumour necrosis factor) inhibitors, 106
tolterodine, 71
toxic chemicals *see* chemicals
trace elements, 77, 83
  plant-based diet and, 132, 133
trans fats, 81
transient global amnesia, 67
transient ischaemic attacks (TIA), 29–31, 145, **214**
trauma, 20–25, 96–99
  personal history, 96–99
  physical *see* injury

psychological/mental, 20, 24–25, 97–99
tuberculosis, 100
tumour necrosis factor (TNF) inhibitors, 106
twin studies and exercise, 148–149

UK *see* United Kingdom
ultra-processed food, eating less, 140–141
uncertainty, living with, x–xi
United Kingdom (UK)
  drugs licensed, 59
  drugs not licensed, 59, 61–62
  NHS *see* NHS
United States of America (US), drugs licensed, 59, 61
urinary infections, 35–36, 36
USA, drugs licensed, 59, 61

vaping, 162
vascular damage (and vascular events) in brain, 23, 24, 26
vascular dementia, 23–24, 26, 29, 145–146, **213**
  AD and, blurred distinction, 24
  diabetes and, 31
  exercise and, 145–146
  genetics, 95
  homocysteine and, 84
  smoking and, 45–46
  stroke and/or transient ischaemic attacks and, 26, 29–31
  subcortical, 30, 104
  types, 29–30
vegan diet, 74, 132, 133
vegetarian diet, 82, 132, 133, 134
vision and falls, 164

Index

Note: AD is the abbreviation for Alzheimer's disease. Glossary page numbers are in bold.

Also from Hammersmith Health Books...

When the Time Comes
Stories from the end of life

Edited by Magnolia Cardona and Ebony Lewis

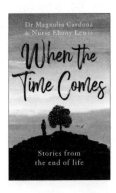

Jointly written and curated by a doctor and a nurse working in end-of-life care, this collection of personal experiences from families and health practitioners throws light on what may be wanted but go unrecognised until it is too late when a loved one or patient is dying. In particular, these stories throw light on the issue of futile over-treatment getting in the way of a peaceful chance to say good-bye.

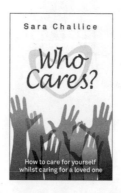

Also from Hammersmith Health Books...

Curing the Incurable
Beyond the limits of medicine

by Dr Jerry Thompson

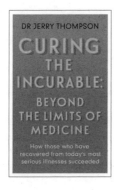

Dr Jerry Thompson draws on an immense range of case
histories and research studies to show how what we eat, the
toxic load we carry, the environmental electromagnetic fields
we live in, and our beliefs and attitudes to health and illness can
change the course of disease. The result is this practical guide to
what we can learn from 'survivors' of 'terminal' illnesses about
how to improve our chances of good health and recovery.

The 'D' Word
Rethinking Dementia

by Mary Jordan and Dr Noel Collins

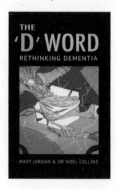

The premise of The 'D' Word is that dementia is here to stay
and a simple cure is very unlikey. But if we rethink it as a social
rather than a purely medical problem we can learn to live
with it rather than fear it, to come to terms with it and gain the
experise needed to manage the many problems it brings.